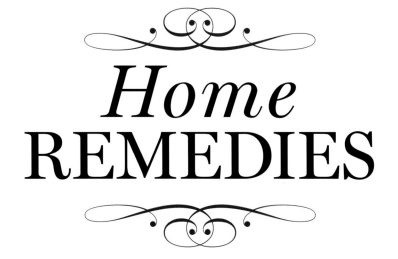

Home
REMEDIES

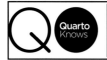

Quarto is the authority on a wide range of topics.

Quarto educates, entertains and enriches the lives of our readers—enthusiasts and lovers of hands-on living.

www.quartoknows.com

First published in the United States of America in 2015 by
Wellfleet Press, a member of
Quarto Publishing Group USA Inc.
142 West 36th Street, 4th Floor
New York, New York 10018
quartoknows.com
Visit our blogs at quartoknows.com

10 9 8 7 6 5 4 3 2

ISBN: 978-1-57715-113-5

Design and Page Layout: Ashley Prine, Tandem Books
Editor: Katherine Furman, Tandem Books
Cover Image: © Sebastian Duda/Shutterstock

Printed in China

The publisher cannot guarantee the accuracy, adequacy, or completeness of the information contained in this book and must disclaim all warranties, expressed or implied, regarding the information. The publisher also cannot assume any responsibility for use of this book, and any use by a reader is at the reader's own risk. This book is not intended to be a substitute for professional medical advice, and any user of this book should always check with a licensed physician before adopting any particular course of treatment or beginning any new health program.

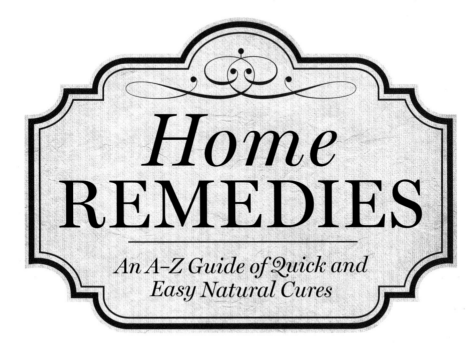

Home
REMEDIES

*An A–Z Guide of Quick and
Easy Natural Cures*

Meredith Hale

WELLFLEET
P R E S S

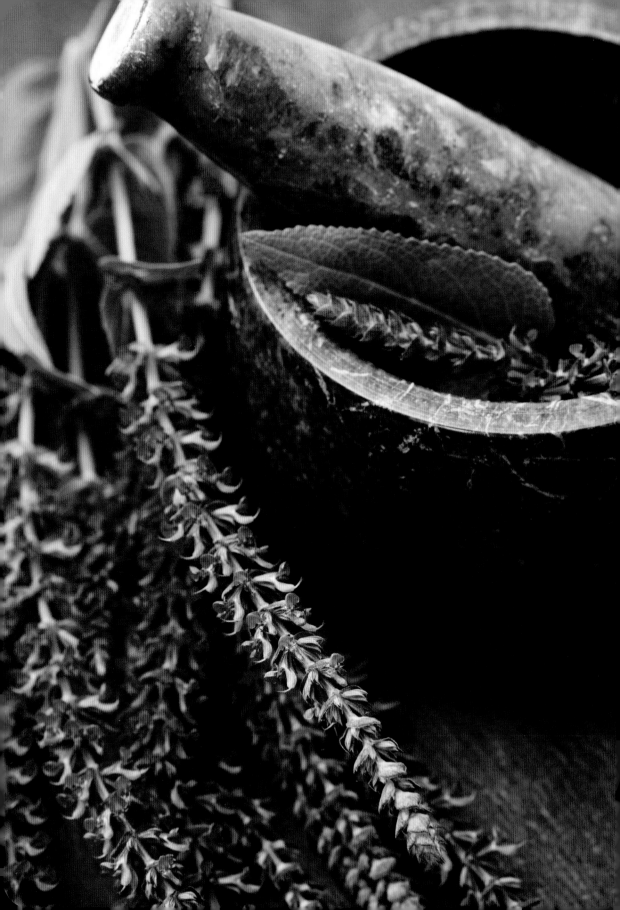

CONTENTS

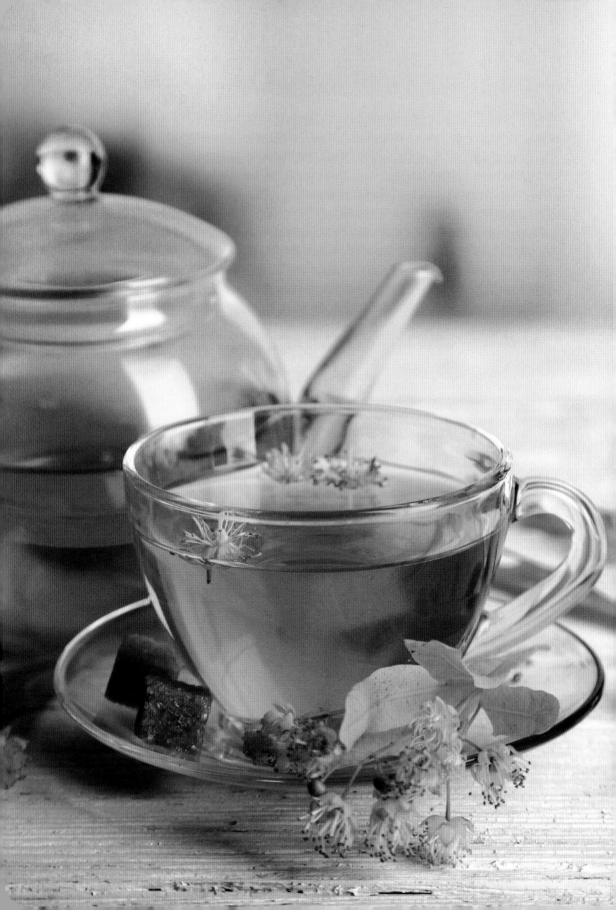

INTRODUCTION

When it comes to treating illnesses, humans have a long history of using the vast resources around them. The Chinese have been enjoying the medicinal benefits of tea for almost five thousand years, ever since a camellia leaf randomly blew into Emperor Shen Nung's cup of hot water. Ancient Greeks and Romans used lemon balm to treat wounds. And Hippocrates himself recommended willow bark for pains and fever—long before its active ingredient, salicin, inspired the creation of aspirin.

In this book is a collection of hundreds of remedies for common health issues, ranging from boils to headaches to shin splints and more. Some are plant-based or herbal remedies used since ancient times to relieve pain and promote healing. Others are "kitchen cures," straight out of your refrigerator or pantry. And still others are in the form of supplements readily available at your local health-food store. While some are "folk cures" your grandmother may have used, others may be less expected. For example, inside these pages you'll learn how to use:

- A tennis ball to eliminate snoring.
- Raw potatoes to relieve eyestrain.
- Socks soaked in egg whites to lower a fever.
- Coconut oil to shrink and relieve hemorrhoids.
- Peppermint to ease irritable bowel syndrome.

If you're new to natural remedies, know that you're joining a large and global community. According to the World Health Organization, nonconventional medicine—which it refers to as traditional and complementary medicine—is found in almost every country in the world, with demand for its services increasing. In the United States, according to the 2012 National Health Interview Survey, more than 33 percent of adults have used complementary health approaches, with fish oil being the top natural health product for adults. Around the world, there is strong interest in new—or, in some cases, ancient—approaches to treating common problems.

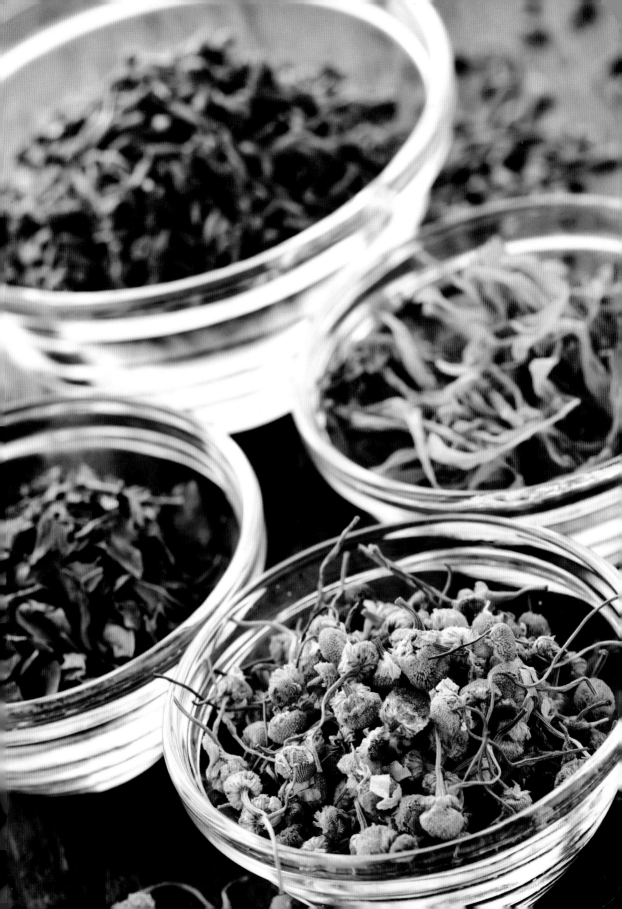

HOME REMEDY SUPERSTARS

As you read these pages, you'll discover that certain remedies come up again and again. That's because certain plants and kitchen cures are used to treat a wide variety of ailments, because they have natural anti-inflammatory and/or antimicrobial properties. ("Antimicrobial" refers to medicines that fight microorganisms, such as bacteria, fungi, and viruses.) Here are just a few of the repeat remedies in this book:

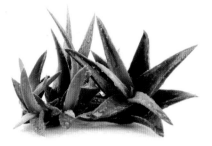

Aloe Vera

Aloe vera's history dates back six thousand years to ancient Egypt, where it was presented as a burial gift to deceased pharaohs. Historically used to heal wounds and treat skin conditions, today aloe vera gel is found in hundreds of skincare products, including sunblocks and after-sun lotions.

Apple Cider Vinegar

Is there anything apple cider vinegar *can't* treat? Also known as ACV, this popular ingredient in salad dressings and marinades is used for ailments as diverse as acne, dandruff, food poisoning, heartburn, jock itch, kidney stones, psoriasis, and more. Cheap and easily accessible, ACV has antibacterial, antifungal, and antiviral properties that make it a staple in any home-remedy arsenal.

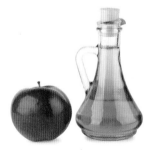

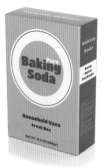

Baking Soda

Sodium bicarbonate—also known as baking soda—does more than just freshen up your refrigerator. Used by ancient Egyptians in its natural form as a cleansing agent, baking soda has a number of contemporary medicinal uses, including treating body odor, poison ivy, calluses, heartburn, and the itching of chickenpox.

Garlic

Garlic has been used medicinally for thousands of years, and today it is used to treat ailments including high blood pressure, high cholesterol, and heart disease. It's also thought to have natural antibiotic and antifungal properties.

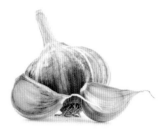

Tea Tree Oil

Used medicinally for centuries by the aboriginal people of Australia, tea tree oil is a common remedy for acne, athlete's foot, nail fungus, wounds, lice, and lots of other ailments.

These and many other home remedies appear repeatedly throughout the book, making it easy to stock up on a few essential items that can treat various ailments you or your family may encounter.

ALWAYS CONSULT YOUR DOCTOR

Home remedies are never a substitute for medical advice from your physician. For starters, many natural treatments and home remedies are not regulated by the Food and Drug Administration (FDA), meaning the regulatory agency has not deemed them safe or effective, or studied their potential side effects. The FDA does regulate dietary supplements, but under a different set of regulations than those covering conventional food and drug products. These regulations place the burden of ensuring safety on the firm manufacturing or distributing the supplement; in fact, dietary supplements do not need approval from the FDA before they are marketed to the public. Therefore, it's important to discuss any potential medical treatments—natural or otherwise—with a medical professional before using them. Here are a few other considerations when evaluating natural treatments for use:

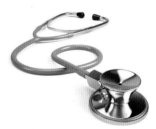

Dosage

Unless otherwise indicated, the dosages recommended here are for adults. Always consult your child's doctor before giving him or her any supplements or other medical treatments. Certain plants or oils can be dangerous for children—for example, peppermint oil should never be given to an infant or very young child, and children under two should not consume honey. The dosages listed here are taken from scientific studies, university and government websites, manufacturer recommendations, and health books; however, as scientific research in this area is often inconsistent, based on small studies, or in need of further corroboration, effective dosages are often hard to pinpoint. Talk to your doctor or a licensed naturopathic doctor (ND) about what's right for you. In addition, keep oils, supplements, and other medicines out of the reach of children, as certain products (such as tea tree oil) may be toxic if ingested or used improperly.

Pregnant and Breastfeeding Women

If you are pregnant or breastfeeding, you should always talk to your doctor before taking any vitamin, supplement, or other medicine (natural or over-the-counter), to make sure it poses no danger to the fetus or baby.

Potential Interactions

If you are currently taking any drugs, or have allergies or other medical conditions, talk to your doctor before beginning a supplement, essential oil, or other treatment. Your doctor can advise you as to potential interactions or side effects. For example:

- Chamomile tea may trigger symptoms in people with allergies to ragweed.
- Cranberries may interfere with blood thinners and other medications.
- Lysine supplements may increase cholesterol production, which can be problematic for people with high cholesterol.

A physician or licensed ND can help you make decisions that take into account your whole body and medical history, and help you avoid potentially dangerous interactions. There is a common misconception that natural and conventional medicines are at odds. In fact, often they can work together. Doctors frequently recommend natural cures for medical problems—for example, an oatmeal bath for eczema or diaper rash. Even if a condition requires conventional medication, home remedies can often complement the medicine prescribed by your doctor by offering pain relief and helping to fight toxins in the body. To begin, find your ailment within these pages, and read the listed treatments and tips. Relief may be as close as your kitchen.

CAUTIONS FOR COMMON HOME REMEDIES

While home remedies are natural and generally very safe, you should always be sure you are using them correctly. For example, many topical remedies are not meant to be ingested. Others may cause allergic reactions in some people or interfere with medications you are already taking. Here is a list of warnings you should understand about some common remedies in this book. As this list is not exhaustive, make sure to discuss with your doctor any supplements or treatments you're considering.

Tea Tree Oil
Make sure never to ingest tea tree oil, as it can be toxic if swallowed. Some people may be allergic to tea tree oil, so test the oil first on a small area of skin, such as the back of the hand. Do don't let your child handle the oil.

Chamomile Tea
Chamomile tea may trigger symptoms in people with allergies to ragweed. Be sure to talk to your doctor if you have any allergies before drinking herbal teas.

Zinc
Talk to your doctor before taking zinc, especially as a nasal spray, as these sprays may be linked to permanent loss of smell.

Honey
Avoid giving honey to children under two years of age, as it may cause infant botulism.

Peppermint
Do not give peppermint tea or oil to an infant or young child, as the menthol it contains can be harmful. Consult your doctor before taking peppermint if you suffer from heartburn or reflux.

Cranberries
Cranberries may interfere with blood thinners and other medications. Talk to your doctor before beginning a supplement if you're taking medication.

❧ ACNE ❧

As long as there have been mirrors, there have been teenagers and adults eager to rid themselves of acne. Acne occurs when pores on the skin become clogged by oil and dead skin cells. It is often triggered by hormonal changes—such as those occurring during adolescence, pregnancy, or around the menstrual cycle—that cause the skin to produce more oil. Certain cosmetics and skin products may also trigger acne. While generally harmless, acne can cause embarrassment and affect a person's self-esteem. Over-the-counter treatments for mild-to-moderate acne include benzoyl peroxide and salicylic acid. More severe cases of acne may be treated by a dermatologist.

If you're looking to save money and avoid potentially harsh chemicals, you can find various remedies right in your kitchen.

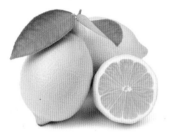

Lemons

Lemon juice destroys the bacteria that cause acne. It also exfoliates the skin and calms inflammation. Before going to bed, apply lemon juice to the affected area with a cotton ball. You can dilute the juice with water to prevent stinging. When you wake up, wash your face following your normal routine.

Tea Tree Oil

Tea tree oil naturally unclogs pores and fights bacteria. Dilute the oil, using a ratio of one part oil to nine parts water. If you find this makes your skin too dry, you can mix a couple drops of tea tree oil in 2–3 teaspoons of aloe vera instead. Use a cotton ball or swab to apply the oil to the acne several times a day.

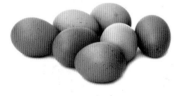

Egg Whites

The proteins in eggs can help to dry out pimples and rebuild skin cells. To use this treatment, first separate the egg whites from the yolks of a few eggs. Whisk the egg whites, and use a cotton ball to cover your face in an egg-white mask. After about half an hour, rinse off the mask with warm water and moisturize your skin.

Apple Cider Vinegar (ACV)

Apple cider vinegar fights bacteria, balances your skin's pH levels, and acts as an astringent, helping to dry up excess oil. To use, first wash your skin with soap and water, and then dry. Dilute the vinegar, using three parts water to one part ACV. (It's important to dilute the vinegar to prevent burning.) Using a cotton ball, apply the mixture to the blemish. After it's dried, wash your skin and apply moisturizer. Repeat this process several times a day.

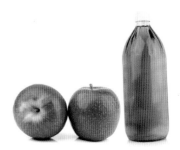

THE LONGTERM

By improving your diet and getting the right vitamins and nutrients, you can improve the overall health of your skin, which means fewer breakouts. Here is a list of what you should make sure you're getting if you want a better complexion:

- **Vitamin A** helps get rid of dead skin cells that build up in pores and cause zits.

- **Zinc** is full of antioxidants and acts as an anti-inflammatory. It also helps metabolize other nutrients.

- **Omega-3 fatty acids** reduce inflammation, which is the core of acne breakouts.

Whether you take supplements or balance your overall diet, getting the recommended daily values of these vitamins and nutrients will not only help clear up acne, it'll promote better health overall.

⋎ ALLERGIES ⋎

Allergies occur when your immune system overreacts to substances that most people's bodies find harmless, such as pollen, ragweed, or dust. Symptoms can include sneezing, itchy eyes, and rashes, among other, more serious reactions. Allergies may be triggered by food, medications, or matter absorbed through the skin or air, such as detergents or pet dander. Common treatments for allergy symptoms include over-the-counter antihistamines and prescription nasal sprays. Severe allergies should be managed by a doctor, and may require lifestyle changes and medication.

Minor allergy symptoms can be treated with easy-to-find plants and oils, as well as some simple modifications in the home.

Nettle

Also referred to as "stinging nettle," this plant functions as a natural antihistamine that can be taken as a tea or in capsule form. To make the tea, place the herb in a mug, pour boiling water over it, and steep for five minutes. Capsules of the freeze-dried leaf can be found in health food stores; take 300 milligrams twice a day.

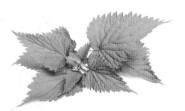

Flaxseed Oil

Flaxseeds are rich in omega-3 fatty acids, which help to reduce inflammatory responses. Flaxseed is available in capsule form, or you can add 1 tablespoon of flaxseed oil daily to a cold beverage such as juice.

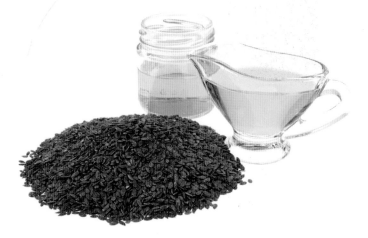

FIGHT THE MITES!

One of the most common triggers for allergy sufferers is dust mites. Dust mites are tiny insects residing in house dust, and the fecal matter they leave on bedding, carpets, and upholstery can plague allergy sufferers year-round. To ease the distress caused by these bugs, try these tips:

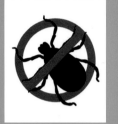

- **Air condition your home.** This both lowers the humidity and filters the air in your home, making it less hospitable to dust mites.

- **Use a dehumidifier.** Again, dust mites thrive in humid air. Keeping your home dry will greatly reduce the dust mite problem in your home.

- **Change your sheets frequently.** Washing your sheets in hot water will help kill the mites.

- **Vacuum carpets and rugs**. Use a model with a high-efficiency particulate air (HEPA) filter, and consider hardwood floors or tile if possible.

While dust mites may seem to be all around you, with a little work, it's possible to fight back, get some relief, and make yourself more comfortable in your own home.

❧ ANXIETY ❧

Everyone experiences anxiety from time to time. It's perfectly natural to get nervous before giving a presentation or taking a big exam, for example. There are many symptoms of anxiety, including lack of concentration, trouble sleeping, irritability, and negative thoughts. While a certain amount of anxiety is normal, anxiety disorders occur when constant fear and worry begin to interfere with a person's daily life. People with anxiety disorders may experience panic attacks, phobias, and excessive worry that keep them from functioning in their work or personal life. While anxiety disorders may require professional care and medication, the occasional bout of anxiety can be calmed with simple remedies such as meditation, herbs, and soothing teas.

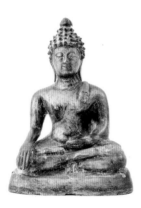

Meditation

Archaeologists have discovered evidence of meditation dating as far back as 5,000 to 3,500 BCE. Meditation can lower blood pressure, improve concentration, and reduce physical and emotional reactions to stress—all of which reduces anxiety. There are many ways to meditate. To start, sit on a chair with your back straight and your feet flat on the floor, your arms on your thighs with your palms turned upward. (Or, you can assume the traditional lotus position.) Breathe regularly by inhaling for six to eight counts, and then holding and exhaling to the same count. Follow these steps daily, gradually increasing the duration of your practice.

Teas

Catnip is a dried herb that acts as a mild sedative. Chamomile is another favorite for soothing frazzled nerves. In 2009, researchers at the University of Pennsylvania found that patients with mild-to-moderate general anxiety disorder who took chamomile supplements reported less anxiety than those on the placebo. Both herbs can be taken in the form of anxiety-relieving teas.

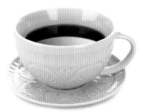

Valerian

If anxiety is keeping you up at night, valerian might help you get the rest you need. A natural sedative, this herb can be taken as a capsule or tincture. To relieve anxiety, take 250 milligrams twice a day; for insomnia, take 270–450 milligrams before you go to sleep.

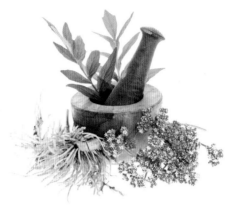

LIFESTYLE MATTERS

If you're suffering from anxiety, these simple lifestyle changes can help:

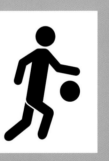

- **Exercise.** Daily cardiovascular activity (twenty to thirty minutes) can trigger the release of feel-good endorphins, improve your self-esteem, and give you a more positive outlook.

- **Limit your alcohol and caffeine intake.** In studies, both have been linked to anxiety.

- **Take a break.** Indulge in soothing silence when you can throughout the day: turn off your phone, step away from the television, or have lunch at the park instead of at your desk.

❧ ARTHRITIS AND JOINT PAIN ❧

Joint stiffness and pain—whether in your hands, knees, hips, or elsewhere—can make it difficult to move and can interfere with your quality of life. If you frequently experience joint pain, you may have arthritis—and if so, you're not alone. According the Centers for Disease Control and Prevention, one in five Americans has been diagnosed with arthritis. Arthritis includes more than one hundred diseases and conditions, the most common of which is osteoarthritis, which causes pain and swelling in the joints, typically in the hands, knees, and spine. Typical treatments include physical therapy, drugs such as NSAIDs like as Advil and Motrin, and sometimes surgery. However, certain anti-inflammatory herbs and other natural approaches can offer relief for arthritis and joint pain.

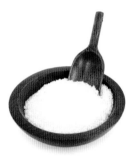

Epsom Salt Bath

Epsom salt is made up of the naturally occurring minerals magnesium and sulfate. Magnesium relaxes muscles, eases pain, and is necessary for the growth and maintenance of bones. For a relaxing bath, add 2 cups of Epsom salt to a tub of warm water and soak for fifteen minutes. You can also eat foods rich in magnesium, such as dark leafy greens, nuts, and beans.

A WEIGHTY MATTER

Did you know that shedding pounds can ease the pain of arthritis? Being overweight adds extra pressure to your joints, burdening your knees, ankles, and hips each time you take a step. Losing weight will help you feel great—inside and out!

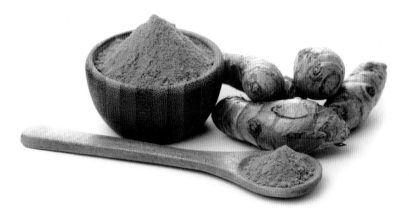

Turmeric

A yellow spice commonly used in Indian cuisine, turmeric and its active compound, curcumin, may reduce inflammation in the body—a big help with arthritis. Make a soothing tea by adding ½ cup each of turmeric and ginger to 2 cups of boiling water. Reduce to a simmer for ten minutes and then strain.

Cinnamon

Another spice with anti-inflammatory properties, cinnamon tastes great while reducing swelling in the body. Sprinkle it on coffee or tea, or on top of other foods and beverages.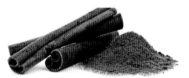

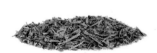 ## Willow Bark

Willow bark has been used since the days of Hippocrates (400 BCE), when patients would chew on it to relieve pain and inflammation. It contains salicin, a chemical similar to aspirin. To make tea from the dried herb, boil 1–2 teaspoons of dried bark in 8 ounces of water; simmer for ten to fifteen minutes and let it steep for half an hour. Drink 3–4 cups daily.

❧ ASTHMA ❧

According to the World Health Organization, 235 million people suffer from asthma worldwide. The most common chronic disease affecting children, asthma occurs when the lining of the bronchial tubes becomes inflamed, narrowing the airways and making it difficult to breathe. Triggers may include allergens such as pollen or dust mites, cigarette smoke, air pollution, or even cold air. Asthma sufferers often rely on medical treatments such as rescue inhalers or anti-inflammatory drugs to reduce tightness and swelling in the airways. To breathe easier on a daily basis, you may also wish to try one of these natural approaches.

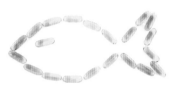

Fish Oil

The omega-3 fatty acids found in certain fish, such as sardines, tuna, and mackerel, have anti-inflammatory properties and may reduce reactions to various allergens that can trigger attacks. Add two servings of fish a week to your diet (plant-based sources such as tofu or walnuts are also beneficial), or add fish oil capsules to your supplement regimen. Recommended dosages vary widely, so consult a doctor on the appropriate amount of DHA and EPA to take, especially for children.

Flavonoids

Flavonoids are compounds found in certain fruits and vegetables that give them their bright colors. They possess antioxidant and antiallergic traits, strengthen capillary walls, and fight inflammation. Add two servings of foods rich in these compounds daily, including apples, onions, tomatoes, and garbanzo beans.

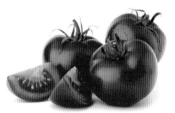

Magnesium

Magnesium may help to relieve muscle tension in the upper respiratory tract. In fact, asthmatics often show low levels of magnesium. Magnesium is found in various foods, such as dark leafy greens, nuts, and beans, or you can take supplements (600 milligrams a day).

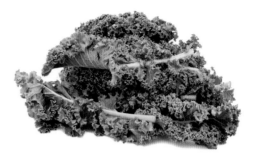

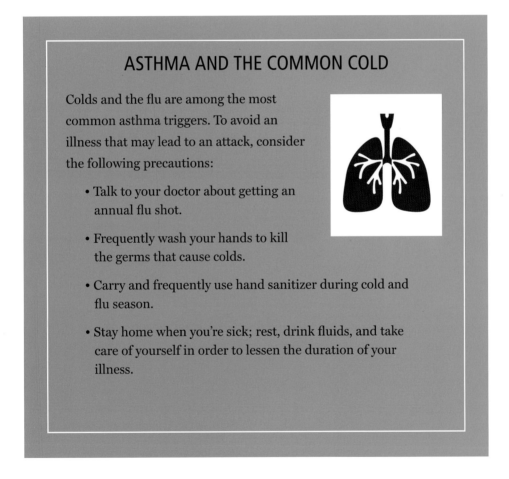

ASTHMA AND THE COMMON COLD

Colds and the flu are among the most common asthma triggers. To avoid an illness that may lead to an attack, consider the following precautions:

- Talk to your doctor about getting an annual flu shot.

- Frequently wash your hands to kill the germs that cause colds.

- Carry and frequently use hand sanitizer during cold and flu season.

- Stay home when you're sick; rest, drink fluids, and take care of yourself in order to lessen the duration of your illness.

❧ ATHLETE'S FOOT ❧

Athlete's foot is a fungal skin infection causing an itchy, irritating rash, typically between the toes. You don't have to be a marathon runner to catch athlete's foot. All you need is contact with a contaminated surface—such as a locker-room floor or the area around a pool, where people typically walk around barefoot. Combine this exposure with tight, sweaty footwear, and you have a recipe for infection. Treating athlete's foot can take time, and often involves over-the-counter antifungal creams or a prescription oral antifungal. When it comes to athlete's foot, an ounce of prevention is worth a pound of cure; however, if you do find yourself in this uncomfortable situation, there are some natural treatments you can turn to for relief.

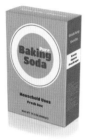

Baking Soda

Baking soda kills bacteria and can act as an antifungal. Mix a tablespoon of baking soda with water to form a paste, and rub on the affected area. Once the paste dries, rinse it off and dry your feet completely with a towel. Sprinkling a little baking soda in your shoes can prevent the moisture in which fungus breeds.

PROPER FOOT CARE

Certain people are more prone to athlete's foot than others. If you find yourself in this category, it's important to watch what you put on your feet. Change your socks often, wash them in hot water, and make sure to wear properly fitting footwear, ideally made of a natural material such as leather.

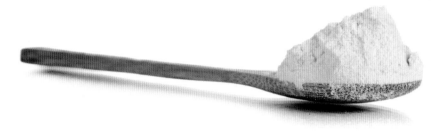

Cornstarch

Cornstarch absorbs moisture, and keeping feet dry is critical to keeping fungus at bay. Brown ½ cup cornstarch in the oven or on the stovetop, making sure it doesn't burn. Rub the cornstarch on your feet and leave it on for five to ten minutes before removing with a towel.

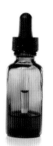

Tea Tree Oil

Considered a natural antiseptic, tea tree oil is active against many bacteria and fungi. Create a mixture of 50 percent tea tree oil and 50 percent olive oil, and rub the combination on the affected area twice a day.

Mouthwash

While mouthwash may not help if you already have athlete's foot, it *can* help to prevent the infection. Mouthwash containing alcohol has antimicrobial properties, reducing bacteria and warding off fungal infections. After each shower, rub a mouthwash-soaked cotton ball on the soles of your feet and between your toes, and allow to dry.

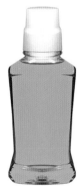

❧ BACK PAIN ❧

Everyone experiences back pain from time to time. This pain can be caused by a sports injury, poor posture, or strain from carrying a heavy weight or strenuous activity. As we grow older, pain can be caused by arthritis or a condition known as intervertebral disc degeneration, in which the discs between the vertebrae of the spine wear down over time. Treatments for debilitating back pain may include physical therapy, chiropractic adjustments, and, as a last resort, surgery. But for a minor sprain or a pulled muscle, some basic home remedies may do the trick.

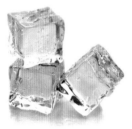

Ice

Ice packs are a simple and effective way to relieve back pain, and, if applied within the first hour or so of an injury, can help to reduce inflammation. Wrap an ice pack in a cloth and hold it on the affected area for fifteen minutes. Repeat every two to three hours. Take care not to place the ice directly on your skin.

Heat

After a couple of days, once the swelling has subsided, try using heat to stimulate circulation and relax sore or knotted muscles. You can apply heat with a heating pad, or take a warm bath. Some people find relief by alternating ice and heat.

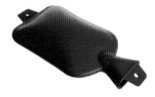

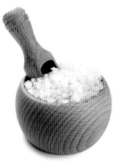

Epsom Salt

Epsom salt is rich in magnesium, which relaxes muscles and eases pain. Add 2 cups of Epsom salt to your bath and soak for half an hour.

GET REST—BUT DON'T OVERDO IT

You need rest to heal a sore or strained back. But if you lie in bed for more than a day or two, you may actually set back your recovery. Engage in moderate movement such as stretching, yoga, or swimming to stay active without further stressing your back muscles. Avoid rigorous activities that involve lifting, bending, or pushing.

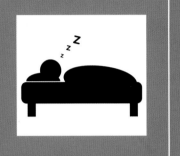

Chamomile Tea

Calming chamomile tea can soothe tense, knotted muscles. To make this tea, steep a tablespoon of chamomile flowers in a mug of boiling water for fifteen minutes. Drink 1–3 cups a day as long as the pain persists.

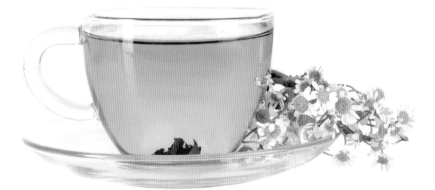

❧ BAD BREATH ❧

Bad breath can ruin a date, distract a colleague, or put off a new acquaintance. Yet for some people, bad breath is a constant fact of life, no matter how diligent their dental hygiene. Bad bread, or halitosis, can be caused by many factors, including eating foods with strong odors, smoking, or bacterial growth between the teeth, around the gums, or on the tongue. Medical causes may include dry mouth, gum disease, yeast infections of the mouth, cavities, and more serious conditions. If you've brushed your teeth, only to discover later your breath is still not sparkling, try these simple solutions.

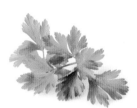

Parsley

Parsley doesn't just dress up your dinner. It also contains chlorophyll, which fights germs and freshens the breath. Chew on some sprigs of parsley or run them through a juicer whenever you want some odor-fighting power.

THINK BEFORE YOU DRINK

You may feel you can't get through the day without your morning cup of coffee—but it may be ruining your breath. The caffeine in coffee can slow saliva production and dry out your mouth, allowing odor-producing bacteria to 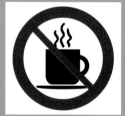 flourish. Coffee also contains sulfur compounds, another culprit behind bad breath. The solution? Replace your morning cup of joe with a brisk jog or a yogurt-based fruit smoothie to get yourself moving in the morning.

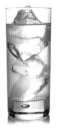

Water

Rinsing with water can moisturize a dry mouth and dislodge bacteria-attracting food particles stuck between the teeth. Drink plenty of water throughout the day, and swish water around your mouth whenever you're experiencing bad breath.

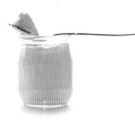

Yogurt

Yogurt contains live bacteria, which may reduce odor-causing bacteria in the mouth, as well as lower levels of hydrogen sulfide, plaque, and gingivitis—all causes of bad breath. To tame bad breath, eat 6 ounces of yogurt a day, preferably plain yogurt without a lot of added sugar.

Cinnamon

Cinnamon has antiseptic properties, and tastes great too! According to research, an essential oil in this spice can kill bacteria in the mouth. Suck on a cinnamon stick or add cinnamon to tea whenever you need to freshen your breath.

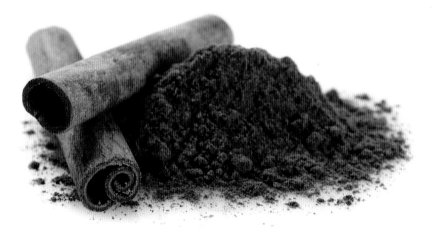

⌁ BLISTERS ⌁

Walking in new shoes, hiking long distances, jogging without socks—all of these can lead to painful blisters, or fluid-filled bumps on the skin. Blisters form when friction causes pockets of fluid to build up between the layers of skin, and are typically found on the hands or feet. Unless caused by an underlying medical condition, blisters are generally harmless and can be cared for at home, using simple treatments.

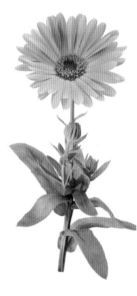

Calendula

The calendula flower reduces pain and swelling. Apply calendula ointment to the blister and cover with a bandage. Allow the blister to air out at night by removing the bandage at bedtime.

WARNING

Do not ingest or use calendula topically if you are pregnant or breastfeeding, or if you are allergic to ragweed, marigolds, or other related plants. Talk to your doctor about your allergies before taking calendula.

Aloe Vera

The healing properties of aloe vera aren't just for sunburns. This plant can also soothe and heal blisters as well. Apply fresh gel from an aloe vera plant to the wound and cover with a bandage or gauze. Try to use the plant rather than an over-the-counter gel, which may contain alcohol that can dry the skin.

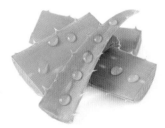

TO DRAIN OR NOT TO DRAIN?

Generally, if a blister is small and not too painful, it's best to leave it alone. The blister's natural covering helps to protect it from bacteria and infection. If the blister is large, painful, or in a spot where it's likely to pop on its own, you may want to consider draining it. Make sure first to sterilize the needle, by holding it over a flame and then letting it cool. After you've punctured and drained the blister, apply an antiseptic ointment and cover it with a bandage. Never pop a blister caused by a burn, as it can get infected.

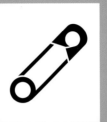

Lavender

With its antibacterial and anti-inflammatory properties, lavender is a great-smelling way to soothe a painful blister. Make a compress by adding a couple drops of lavender essential oil to a glass of cold water. Use a cloth to apply the mixture to the blister for several minutes. Repeat two to three times a day.

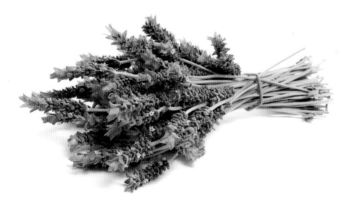

❧ BLOATING ❧

Everyone's experienced it: after a festive holiday dinner or a particularly indulgent night of snacking, your stomach swells and you feel pain or cramping in your belly. Bloating is a buildup of gas in your stomach or intestines. It can be caused by many factors, including overeating, eating fatty or gas-producing foods, drinking carbonated beverages, or stress and anxiety. Severe or chronic bloating may be a sign of a gastrointestinal infection, or may be related to medical conditions such as celiac disease or irritable bowel syndrome. Bloating is often relieved simply by passing gas or a bowel movement. If relief isn't forthcoming, however, try one of these home remedies to win the battle of the bulging belly.

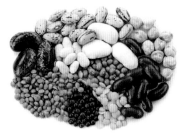

Magnesium

Magnesium can help soothe a troubled digestive system by expelling gas and relieving constipation by relaxing muscles in the walls of the intestines. This mineral is present in foods such as dark leafy greens, nuts, and beans. Or, you can take a magnesium supplement, 200 milligrams a day.

Probiotics

You've probably heard of probiotics and the "good bacteria" they contain that can aid in digestive health. Look for probiotic supplements (in capsule or powder form), or add probiotic-containing foods such as kefir or yogurt to your diet.

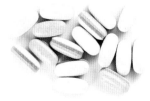

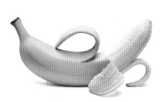

Potassium

Potassium can make you feel less bloated by helping to circulate fluids in the body. Dietary sources of potassium include sweet potatoes, beans, and bananas. Be careful with bananas, however—too many can lead to constipation.

Dandelion Tea

Drink 1 cup of dandelion tea daily to relieve water retention in your body and aid in the breakdown of fatty foods.

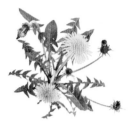

Fiber

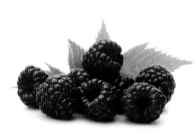

High-fiber foods move quickly through your digestive tract, and can ease constipation and bloating. Foods rich in fiber include whole grains, beans, fruits such as raspberries and pears, and vegetables such as celery, carrots, and broccoli. To keep your digestive system in check, increase your fiber intake gradually, as suddenly increasing dietary fiber may actually worsen your bloating. And, as always, drink plenty of water to keep things moving.

THERE'S AIR IN THERE

Swallowing air can lead to gas in your digestive system—which in turn can lead to bloating. If you have frequent bloating, try cutting back on these "airy" habits:

- Chewing gum or sucking on hard candy

- Drinking carbonated beverages such as soda

- Drinking through a straw

By making a few lifestyle changes, you can improve your digestion and ease the discomfort of bloating.

❧ BODY ODOR ❧

Like bad breath, body odor (or BO) is an embarrassing problem that can affect relationships and shake a person's self-esteem. Ironically, according to some experts, human odors once played a vital part in mating. Today, drugstore shelves are lined with products to manage unwanted odors. If these products aren't working for you, you may want to try a different approach.

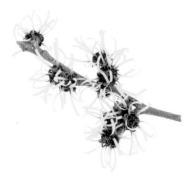

Witch Hazel

If your usual deodorant isn't working, try swapping it for some witch hazel. Body odor occurs when bacteria break down sweat into acids, creating an unpleasant smell. Witch hazel lowers the skin's pH levels, making it difficult for odor-causing bacteria to survive. Apply it to your underarms with a cotton ball as frequently as you would apply deodorant.

WHEN IT'S NOT JUST A SMELL . . .

If you're suddenly sweating more than usual for no apparent reason or you have cold sweats, night sweats, or your sweat smells different than usual, see a doctor to make sure you don't have an underlying cause. Conditions such as hyperthyroidism and diabetes can alter the amount and scent of a person's sweat. A doctor can rule out any such problems and help you get to the bottom of your excessive sweating.

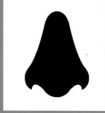

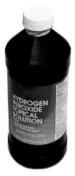

Hydrogen Peroxide

Hydrogen peroxide reduces the amount of bacteria on the skin, allowing less odor. Wipe the hydrogen peroxide onto your underarms as a natural deodorant. You can also use rubbing alcohol or apple cider vinegar for the same purpose, so long as they don't dry out your skin.

Baking Soda and Cornstarch

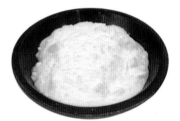

Like hydrogen peroxide, baking soda kills the bacteria that cause odors. In addition, both baking soda and cornstarch absorb moisture such as sweat on the skin. After bathing, apply baking soda or cornstarch directly to your underarms—or, to reduce odor *and* soak up sweat, mix the two together before applying.

Essential Oils

Various essential oils fight bacteria while giving off a pleasant odor. Try applying lavender or peppermint directly to the affected area for a fresh scent. (Do not apply peppermint oil on an infant or young child.) Or, drink these herbs as tea to treat body odor from the inside out.

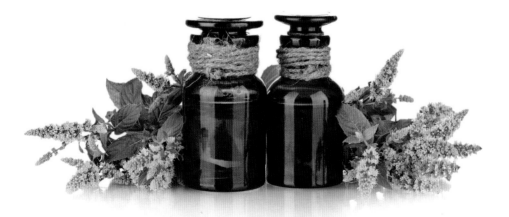

❧ BOILS ❧

A boil forms when staph bacteria enter the skin through a hair follicle, oil gland, or cut. After a few days, pus collects under the skin, and the bump grows larger and more painful, until it eventually ruptures and drains—generally after a couple of weeks. Boils tend to appear on the face, neck, shoulders, armpits, or buttocks; if a boil appears on the eyelid, it's called a sty. To relieve the pain and irritation of a boil, use these natural methods to bring it to a head and speed up the healing process.

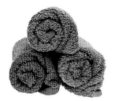

Warm Compress

Heat can help a boil form a head and drain. Soak a washcloth in warm water and apply it to the boil for ten minutes or longer every few hours. Make sure to keep the washcloth as warm as possible during this process.

Bread Poultice

A popular folk remedy, this method works similarly to a warm compress, by bringing the boil to a head and reducing inflammation. Soak a piece of bread in warm water or milk, and apply it directly to the boil for several minutes. Repeat twice a day.

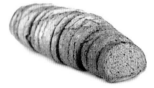

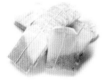

Tea Bags

To reduce the swelling and pain of a boil, apply warm tea bags every one to two hours. Tea bags contain tannins, an astringent that can shrink inflamed tissue.

Acne Cream

Bringing a boil to a head is one way to get rid of it. However, drying it out can eliminate it as well. Apply an acne product with benzoyl peroxide twice a day.

WHEN TO CALL THE DOCTOR

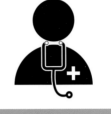

A boil may indicate a more serious condition if it:

- Causes extreme pain

- Lasts longer than two weeks

- Is accompanied by chills or a fever

If any of these conditions are present, see a doctor immediately. Also, avoid squeezing or puncturing the boil yourself, as you may spread the infection.

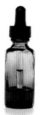

Tea Tree Oil

Fight boils with antibacterial, antiseptic tea tree oil. Dilute the oil by mixing one part oil with nine parts water, so it's gentler on the skin. Use a cotton ball or swab to apply the mixture to the boil several times a day.

Garlic

Garlic has natural antibiotic properties, and can expel toxins from the skin. To use, place crushed, raw garlic on the boil and cover with a bandage.

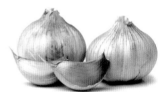

❦ BRUISES ❦

If you're prone to bumps and falls (or just the hazards of everyday life), you probably find yourself with the occasional black-and-blue marks on your skin. Bruises occur when a knock or injury to the body causes small blood vessels under the skin to burst, leading blood to collect under the skin. Bruises generally go away on their own within a couple of weeks, without any treatment. However, if you need to show some skin—and don't want to look like you just went a few rounds in the ring—consider these treatments to speed up the healing process.

Ice

Your mom knew what she was doing when she put frozen peas on your bumps and bruises. Ice compresses serve to reduce swelling and constrict blood vessels, allowing less blood to seep into surrounding tissue. Apply ice or frozen vegetables wrapped in a towel to the bruise as soon as possible, and leave it on for at least fifteen minutes. Repeat this every one to two hours the first twenty-four hours after you receive the bruise.

Warm Compress

Once the frozen veggies are back in the freezer (after the first twenty-four hours), treat the bruise with a warm compress to encourage blood flow. Soak a washcloth in warm water and apply it to the bruise for ten minutes. Repeat a few times a day until the bruise begins to fade.

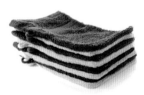

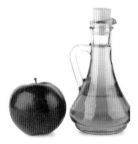

Apple Cider Vinegar

A natural anti-inflammatory, apple cider vinegar can help to heal that bruise quickly. Apply it directly to the bruise with a cotton ball.

Arnica

Arnica comes from a plant that grows in the Rocky Mountains. It has anti-inflammatory properties and dilates the capillaries, moving the blood away from the bruise. Apply arnica gel directly to the bruise, three to four times a day.

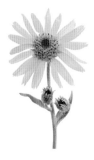

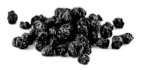

Bilberry Extract

Bilberry extract contains powerful antioxidants that strengthen capillaries and increase vitamin C levels in the cells. Take bilberry extract as a supplement, or if you prefer, consume 20–60 grams of dried berries a day. You can also make a tea using 5–10 grams (1–2 teaspoons) of mashed berries, or steep 1–2 teaspoons of finely chopped dried bilberry leaf in boiling water for five to ten minutes, and then strain.

IF YOU BRUISE EASILY . . .

If you find that you're constantly black and blue, this may be a sign of a vitamin C deficiency. You can add more vitamin C to your diet with fruits and vegetables, or by taking 1 gram of oral vitamin C daily. In some cases, easy bruising can signify a more serious condition, such as a clotting disorder. Be sure to speak to your doctor if you bruise frequently or if your bruises don't heal in a timely manner.

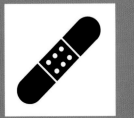

❧ BURNS ❧

Ouch! Whether you inadvertently grabbed a hot pan or spilled coffee on your lap, burns are extremely painful—and can even land you in the emergency room. First-degree burns affect the outer layer of the skin; with second-degree burns, the second layer of skin (the dermis) is burned as well, with blisters and swelling typical. The most severe burns are third-degree burns, which can affect nerves and muscles in addition to the skin, and are charred or white in appearance. First-degree burns and small second-degree burns can be treated at home. For more serious burns or chemical burns, be sure to seek medical attention. (For sunburns, see page 184.)

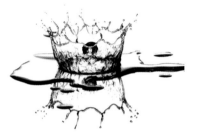

Cool Water

For minor burns, hold the affected area under cool—not cold—water for ten to fifteen minutes, until the burning stops. The cool water reduces swelling and carries the heat away from your skin.

WARNING

Some old wives' tales are dangerous when it comes to burns. Putting ice on a burn can make it worse, and applying butter can cause infection. Try one of the treatments listed here or see a doctor if necessary.

White Vinegar

The acetic acid in white vinegar helps to relieve the pain and inflammation of a burn, and its antiseptic qualities can prevent it from getting infected. Use a cotton ball to dab the burn with white vinegar, or create a compress with diluted vinegar.

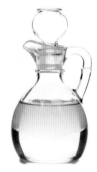

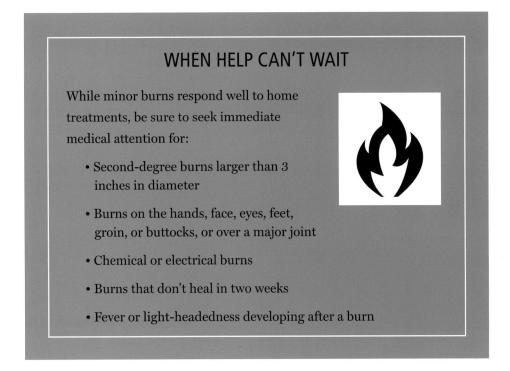

WHEN HELP CAN'T WAIT

While minor burns respond well to home treatments, be sure to seek immediate medical attention for:

- Second-degree burns larger than 3 inches in diameter

- Burns on the hands, face, eyes, feet, groin, or buttocks, or over a major joint

- Chemical or electrical burns

- Burns that don't heal in two weeks

- Fever or light-headedness developing after a burn

Tea Bags

The tannins in black tea can draw heat away from a burn. Apply two to three cool, wet black tea bags to the wound, securing the bags with sterile gauze.

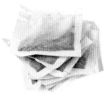

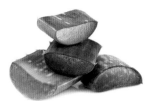

Aloe

Aloe naturally moisturizes the skin and dulls pain, easing the sting of a burn. Place the gel from a fresh aloe leaf directly on the burn.

Coconut Oil

Coconut oil has natural antifungal and antibacterial qualities to help keep your burn from getting infected. It's also rich in vitamin E, an antioxidant that helps to repair and protect the skin. Apply the coconut oil directly to the affected area.

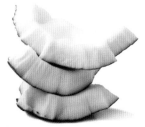

❧ CALLUSES AND CORNS ❧

While they may look unsightly, calluses and corns are actually your body's way of protecting itself. Calluses occur when your skin forms thin, hard layers to protect itself against friction, pressure, and other irritation. They most commonly occur on the feet or the hands. Corns are small patches of hardened, dead skin occurring on the tops, sides, or in between the toes. Common causes of calluses and corns are high heels or tight footwear that leads to rubbing and friction on the feet. While calluses and corns may be unattractive and, in some situations uncomfortable, they are rarely dangerous and often heal on their own. However, if they bother you, try one of these skin-smoothing solutions.

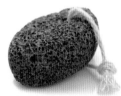

Pumice Stone

Perhaps the fastest way to get rid of dead skin cells is to remove them. After soaking the corn or callused area using one of the below methods, use a pumice stone to slough away the dead skin.

Warm Soak

To soften the skin and loosen dead skin cells, soak the affected area for thirty minutes in warm water containing one of the following:

- **Baking Soda:** Add 3 tablespoons of baking soda to a basin of warm water to break up dead skin cells.
- **Epsom Salt:** Add salt to warm water to scrub away dead cells while softening the skin.
- **Chamomile Tea:** Mixed in warm water, this also will soften hardened skin.

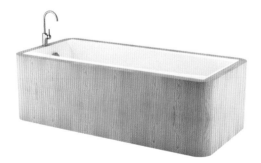

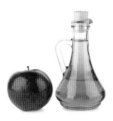

Apple Cider Vinegar

Soak a slice of bread in apple cider vinegar overnight, until it forms a paste. Apply the paste to your callus or corn before going to bed and cover in a plastic wrap. Rinse off the paste in the morning.

Licorice

It's hard to believe, but an estrogen-like substance in licorice may just soften up that hard skin! Grind up three or four licorice sticks, and mix them with ½ teaspoon of either petroleum jelly or sesame oil. Apply this paste to the callus or corn before going to bed.

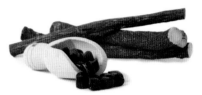

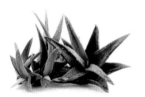

Aloe

Soften your skin with gel from an aloe plant. Use a bandage to adhere an aloe leaf to your callus or corn, with the gel side against the affected area. Leave on overnight.

LOSE THOSE SHOES

The best way to prevent calluses and corns is to ditch those heels or sandals that pinch your feet or cause excess friction. Wear socks when you can, and shop for comfortable, proper-fitting shoes made of natural materials like leather. Save those high heels for a special night on the town—your feet will thank you!

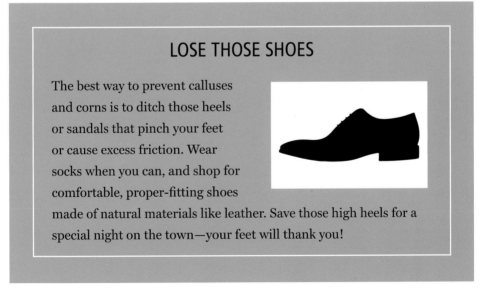

❧ CANKER SORES ❧

A canker sore is a small lesion inside the mouth that can cause pain when talking or eating. Typically found on or under the tongue, inside the lips or cheeks, or on the roof of the mouth, canker sores are often white or yellow with a red border. Unlike cold sores, they are not contagious. Doctors aren't sure exactly what causes canker sores, but they suspect triggers may include injuries from dental work or rigorous brushing, acidic or citrus fruits and vegetables, allergic reactions to bacteria in the mouth, or hormone changes during menstruation, among other causes. Canker sores typically resolve on their own after one or two weeks, although painful sores can be treated with over-the-counter medications, prescription rinses, or medical treatments—as well as simple remedies straight out of your garden or kitchen.

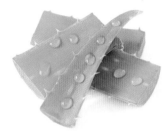

Aloe Vera

The gel from this wonder-plant can dull the pain of uncomfortable canker sores. Squeeze the gel from the leaf and apply it directly to the canker sore with a cotton ball or swab. Repeat several times a day until the pain subsides.

IS IT YOUR TOOTHPASTE?

Could the toothpaste you use to protect your mouth be causing your canker sores? Studies have shown that sodium lauryl sulfate (SLS), a common foaming agent in toothpastes, may contribute to recurrent canker sores. If you're a frequent sufferer, consider switching to a toothpaste without this ingredient.

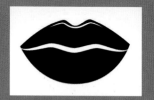

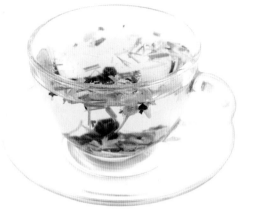

Chamomile Tea

Anti-inflammatory and antiseptic properties found in chamomile tea can reduce the pain of canker sores and promote healing. Soak a teabag in water for one minute and then apply to the affected area for five to ten minutes twice a day.

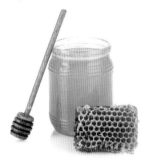

Honey

For sweet relief of painful sores, try a dab of honey. Researchers at Saudi Arabia's Salman bin Abdulaziz University found that patients treated with honey reported quicker pain relief and elimination of sores than those taking a prescription or over-the-counter product. After each meal, wipe the area clean with a wet cotton ball, and then apply honey with a cotton swab.

Yogurt

It's hard to believe that simply eating yogurt can help prevent a canker sore, but the "good" bacteria in yogurt can balance out the "bad" bacteria in the mouth and digestive system. If you're prone to getting canker sores, consider adding 1 cup of yogurt to your daily diet—and make sure the packaging says it contains "live cultures." For a healthier snack, choose plain yogurt and add a little honey for extra sore-fighting power.

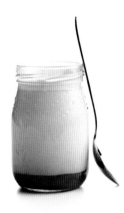

❦ CARPAL TUNNEL SYNDROME ❦

If you frequently experience tingling or numbness in your fingers and hands, or shooting pain in your wrists or forearm, you may have carpal tunnel syndrome. It occurs when the median nerve, which controls sensations in the thumb and fingers (excluding the pinky), becomes compressed in the space in the wrist known as the carpal tunnel. Various factors may contribute to carpal tunnel syndrome, including wrist fractures, chronic illnesses such as diabetes, inflammatory conditions such as arthritis, pregnancy, and lifestyle factors such as performing repetitive tasks involving flexing of the wrist. While many people associate computer use with carpal tunnel syndrome, studies are not conclusive as to this link. Treatments may include wrist splints, medications, and even surgery. If you're experiencing carpal tunnel syndrome, consider these herbal treatments to ease your discomfort and speed your recovery.

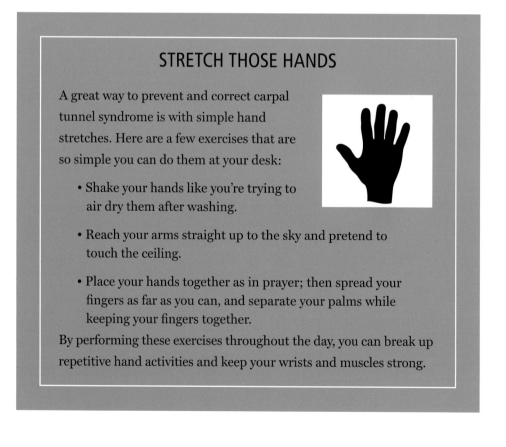

STRETCH THOSE HANDS

A great way to prevent and correct carpal tunnel syndrome is with simple hand stretches. Here are a few exercises that are so simple you can do them at your desk:

- Shake your hands like you're trying to air dry them after washing.

- Reach your arms straight up to the sky and pretend to touch the ceiling.

- Place your hands together as in prayer; then spread your fingers as far as you can, and separate your palms while keeping your fingers together.

By performing these exercises throughout the day, you can break up repetitive hand activities and keep your wrists and muscles strong.

Heat

To relax tightened muscles, try packing some heat. Each night, soak your hands and wrists in hot water for fifteen minutes.

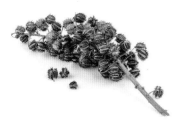

Castor Oil

Castor oil can also fight inflammation, and combined with heat, can provide powerful relief from carpal tunnel syndrome. Apply the castor oil to a cloth and place it on your wrist. Cover the entire area with plastic wrap. Apply a heating pad for an hour. Repeat this process four to five nights a week until the pain subsides.

Arnica

An herbal treatment with anti-inflammatory properties, arnica was shown in a study at the Department of Plastic Surgery of Queen Victoria Hospital in West Sussex, England, to reduce pain after hand surgery, compared to a placebo. Massage a quarter teaspoon of arnica ointment into the wrist twice a day until you experience relief.

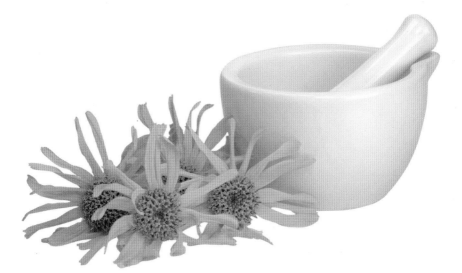

⤜ CHAFING ⤛

Are your clothes rubbing you the wrong way? When skin rubs against skin or clothing, irritation known as skin chafing can occur—making skin red, inflamed, and more susceptible to infection. Chafing is common among the obese, long-distance athletes, and people with sensitive skin, and it's exacerbated by sweat and bacteria on the skin. Chafing most frequently occurs on the thighs, groin, nipples, and underarms, although any part of the body where excess friction occurs can be vulnerable to chafing. If your workout clothes are leaving your skin raw and irritated, go for a more sports-friendly material, and try these soothing remedies to relieve your chafed skin.

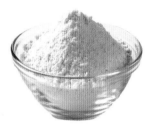

Cornstarch

Since sweat can lead to chafing, it's important to keep the skin dry. Not only does cornstarch absorb moisture, but it also can prevent the growth of fungus in the area. Gently rub cornstarch onto the affected skin as often as necessary. As an alternative, you can sprinkle talcum or baby powder on sweaty areas as well.

Petroleum Jelly

Reducing friction can relieve and eliminate chafing. Rub some petroleum jelly on the chafed area to protect it from further irritation and begin healing.

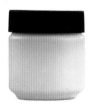

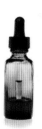

Tea Tree Oil

Tea tree oil protects against infection and fights bacteria on the skin that contributes to chafing. Add a few drops of tea tree oil to an unscented moisturizer and apply to the chafed skin several times a day.

Witch Hazel

With its anti-inflammatory properties, witch hazel can soothe the sting of chafed skin. Apply a cold compress soaked in witch hazel directly to the chafed skin to cool it down and begin healing.

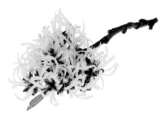

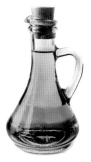

Olive Oil

The moisturizing properties of olive oil make it a potent remedy for chafed skin. Rub olive oil directly on the affected area for relief. Or, combine olive oil with oatmeal to make a paste you can apply to the skin. Leave the paste on for half an hour before washing it off.

Aloe Vera

The gel from an aloe vera plant can relieve the itch and burning of chafed skin. Apply it directly to the skin.

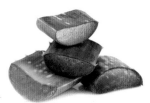

FRICTION-FREE FABRICS

If you're a long-distance runner or biker, or if you typically exercise for long stretches of time, finding the right fabrics is essential to avoid painful chafing. Avoid cotton shirts or sweatpants that get wet and stay wet.

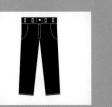

Instead, look for lightweight, synthetic materials that dry quickly. Consider biking shorts to reduce friction on the thighs.

❧ CHAPPED LIPS ❧

Dry, cracked lips are one of the many banes of winter. When the weather turns cold and dry, the thin skin on the lips can suffer. Unfortunately, this dryness instinctively provokes us to lick our lips—further drying them out and exacerbating the problem. While chapped lips aren't dangerous, they can sting, bleed, and even make your lips vulnerable to a cold sore or infection. If your lips have fallen victim to the elements, try these natural suggestions—and kiss chapped lips goodbye.

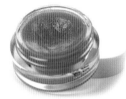

Lip Balm
The key to protecting your lips from the wrath of winter is to moisturize them. You ideally want a moisturizing balm that forms a barrier between your lips and the air. Look for an oil-based balm or apply petroleum jelly throughout the day.

Coconut Oil
With its moisturizing, antibacterial, and antifungal properties, coconut oil is a natural choice for chapped lips. Plus, it smells great! Apply it to your lips as often as necessary.

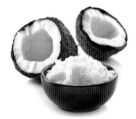

HYDRATION FROM THE INSIDE OUT

When it comes to chapped lips, staying hydrated can be one of your best defenses. Be sure to drink extra water during the winter months, and use a humidifier in your bedroom. Avoid smoking, drinking alcohol, or eating too much salt, as these can dehydrate your body.

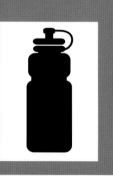

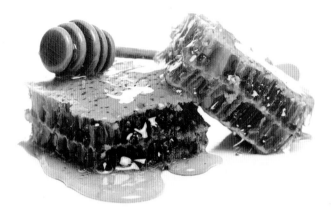

Honey

Honey moisturizes dry skin and has antibacterial properties as well. Rub honey on your chapped lips throughout the day, or make a paste with sugar (see below).

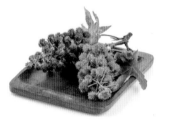

Castor Oil

Castor oil does a great job lubricating dry, chapped lips. Apply castor oil to your lips several times a day, or mix equal parts castor oil and glycerin with a few drops of lemon juice to make a healing treatment you can leave on overnight.

Sugar

Sugar naturally exfoliates the skin, removing the dead skin cells that accompany chapped lips. Mix equal parts sugar and olive oil or honey to form a paste. Rub this paste on your lips to loosen the dead skin; after a few minutes, wipe it off with warm water.

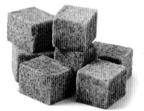

❧ CHICKENPOX ❧

Many adults remember the itchy rash and blisters of chickenpox, or varicella. Until recently, chickenpox was extremely common—according to the Centers for Disease Control and Prevention, before the vaccine, an average of four million people got chickenpox each year in the United States, with the highest incidence in preschool-aged children. Since the vaccine, however, rates of this contagious disease have dropped dramatically. In fact, according to the CDC, varicella declined 82 percent from 2000 to 2010. That means a lot less itching, fewer hospitalizations—and a lot less missed school. For unvaccinated children and adults unlucky enough to catch this itchy illness, several home remedies offer relief while the virus runs its course.

WHEN HOME CARE ISN'T ENOUGH

As a childhood disease, chickenpox has always been considered more of a pain than a peril. However, if you or your child have chickenpox, and any of the below symptoms occur, be sure to call your doctor right away:

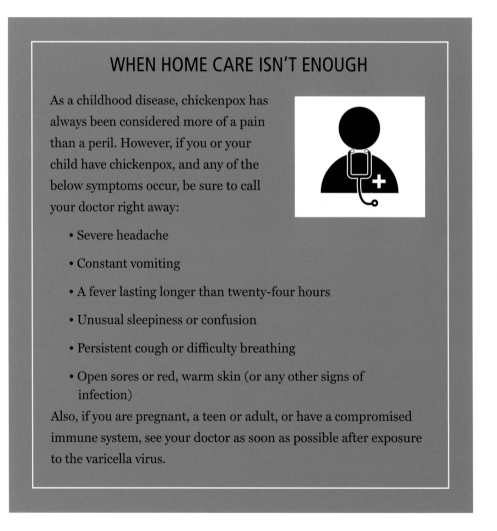

- Severe headache

- Constant vomiting

- A fever lasting longer than twenty-four hours

- Unusual sleepiness or confusion

- Persistent cough or difficulty breathing

- Open sores or red, warm skin (or any other signs of infection)

Also, if you are pregnant, a teen or adult, or have a compromised immune system, see your doctor as soon as possible after exposure to the varicella virus.

Baking Soda

Baking soda can also relieve the itching of varicella. Place ½ to 1 cup baking soda (depending on how full the tub is) in slightly cool water and soak for fifteen to twenty minutes. You can do this every few hours until the itching subsides.

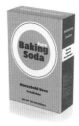

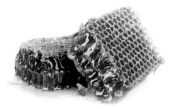

Honey

Honey has antibacterial properties, relieves pain, and may help prevent scarring. Apply a thin layer over the blisters three times a day.

Oatmeal

Oatmeal is known to soothe itchy, irritated skin. Grind 2 cups oatmeal into a powder and pour it into a coffee filter bag or nylon stocking tied off at the end. Place the bag in the back of a warm tub and allow water to cool (as heat can worsen the itch). Soak for fifteen to twenty minutes.

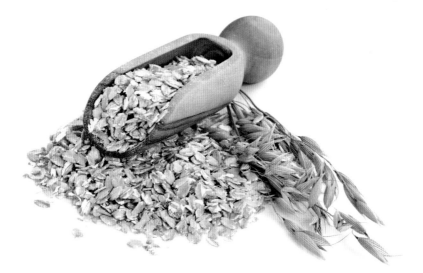

❧ COLD SORES ❧

Also known as fever blisters, cold sores are tiny fluid-filled blisters found around the lips. After a period of time, the blister breaks, oozing fluid and forming a crust. In addition to itching and burning, cold sores may be accompanied by fever, sore throat, and swollen lymph nodes. Cold sores are caused by a strain of herpes simplex virus (HSV), often passed between people through activities such as kissing or sharing towels or utensils. Unfortunately, while the cold sore may subside, there is no cure for HSV once it's in your body; if you've contracted HSV, cold sores may recur in the future. Cold sores usually go away on their own within two weeks; however, to speed healing, there are several alternatives to antiviral pills and creams.

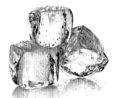

Ice and Cold Water

To help ease the burning and discomfort of cold sores, try applying ice or cold compresses to the affected area. Repeat every few hours until the pain subsides.

Lemon Balm

Ancient Greeks and Romans used topical lemon balm, also called Melissa, to treat wounds. Today it's a popular treatment for both genital and oral herpes, due to its antiviral properties. Studies have shown it to lessen the duration and intensity of cold sores. For active flare-ups, apply a thick layer of lemon balm cream four times a day. To prevent future outbreaks, apply twice a day.

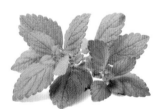

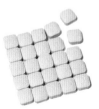

Zinc

Studies in Boston and Israel found zinc to be effective in reducing the length of the herpes outbreak, preventing the virus's DNA from replicating. As soon as a cold sore makes an appearance, dissolve a zinc lozenge (like those used for sore throats) on the lesion.

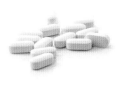

Lysine

This amino acid may inhibit herpes activity and prevent future occurrences. Apply lysine cream to cold sores twice daily or as advised on the label. For prevention, take 500 milligrams a day as a supplement.

WARNING

Be sure to monitor your cholesterol levels while taking lysine supplements, as lysine may increase cholesterol production.

Licorice

With its antiviral and anti-inflammatory properties, licorice can be an effective weapon against cold sores. Mix a tablespoon of licorice root powder or extract with 2 teaspoons of petroleum jelly, and apply the mixture to the cold sore with a cotton swab. Leave on for several hours or overnight.

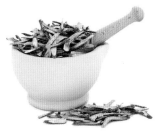

THE STRESS OF COLD SORES

If you suffer from recurring cold sores, stress can be a trigger. To fight stress, practice relaxation techniques such as meditation, yoga, and deep-breathing exercises. Make sure to get plenty of rest and set aside time for friends and loved ones.

❧ COLDS AND FLU ❧

We've all heard the bad news: there's no cure for the common cold. Technically a viral infection of the nose and throat (the upper respiratory tract), colds are the culprit behind the runny noses, coughing, and congestion that plague adults and children throughout the year. Colds are spread through the air when someone coughs or sneezes, or through contact with a contaminated surface, such as a drinking glass or towel. The rhinovirus, the most common of the more than two hundred viruses causing the common cold, is contagious, opportunistic, and no fun to catch. But just because there's no cure, doesn't mean you have to suffer in silence. Fortunately, several natural treatments can relieve your symptoms and speed your path to recovery.

Saltwater Gargle

Saltwater can offer relief to a dry or scratchy throat. Dissolve ¼–½ teaspoon of salt in an 8-ounce glass of warm water and briefly gargle several times a day to soothe your irritated throat.

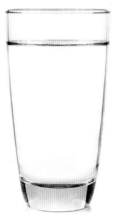

COLD OR FLU?

While they share certain symptoms, influenza and colds are caused by different viruses. Flu symptoms typically include fever, chills, head and body aches, and fatigue—and often the sneezing, runny nose, and sore throat of a cold. Many of the cold remedies listed here can ease flu symptoms as well; in addition, see the chapters on *fatigue*, *fever*, and *headaches* to address these individual symptoms of the flu.

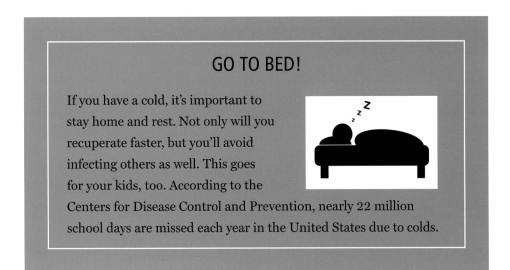

GO TO BED!

If you have a cold, it's important to stay home and rest. Not only will you recuperate faster, but you'll avoid infecting others as well. This goes for your kids, too. According to the Centers for Disease Control and Prevention, nearly 22 million school days are missed each year in the United States due to colds.

Zinc

Zinc has been shown to reduce the duration of a cold, possibly by preventing the rhinovirus from multiplying or from adhering to the mucus membranes of the throat and nose. When a cold rears its head, suck on a zinc gluconate lozenge every few hours. Follow the instructions on the label and do not exceed the recommended dose.

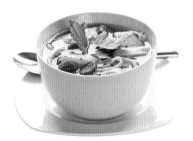

Chicken Soup

According to researchers, this folk remedy really can ease your symptoms. Chicken soup acts as an anti-inflammatory and encourages movement of mucus through the nose, relieving congestion. For an added antiviral punch, add some raw chopped garlic to your bowl. (Raw garlic is preferable for medicinal purposes, as cooking it may destroy the compounds and enzymes that make it effective.)

Vitamin C

Vitamin C may reduce the duration of your cold, as well as relieve some of your coughing and sneezing. The recommended dose is 100 to 500 milligrams a day.

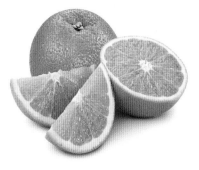

❦ COLIC ❦

Colic is the scourge of new—and exhausted—parents everywhere. Colicky babies often cry for more than three hours a day, for no discernible reason, and no amount of nourishment or cuddling can soothe them. The exact cause of colic is unknown. Scientists attribute it to causes as diverse as reflux, a reaction to lactose in certain formulas, gas, overstimulation, and just plain moodiness. Colic begins in babies around two weeks of age, and generally disappears on its own by the four-month mark. While the situation is temporary, frustrated parents are eager to do anything they can to soothe their colicky child—as quickly as possible. For relief of this condition, try some of these soothing techniques.

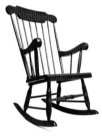

Stomach Position

Approaches connecting colic to tummy trouble focus on soothing a baby's abdomen. To try the "colic carry," position your baby with her body along your forearm, stomach down, her cheek in the palm of your hand and legs straddling your forearm. For added soothing, hold baby in this position while gently rocking back and forth in a rocking chair.

Diet

To test if your baby has a sensitivity to a certain food, breast-feeding mothers can try eliminating common allergens from their diets, such as milk and other dairy products, peanuts, and wheat. Talk to your doctor before making major changes to your diet if you're nursing.

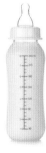

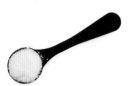

Formula

To see if formula is causing your baby's colic, try switching to hydrolysate infant formula. Whole milk proteins in this formula are already broken down for easier digestion.

Reduce Gas

Some doctors attribute colic to excess gas in a baby's system. If you're bottle-feeding, try holding baby upright during feedings and pause throughout to burp her. Also, try a different bottle or nipple that might allow for less air intake when feeding.

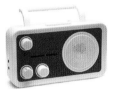

White Noise

Some experts believe that white noise recreates the atmosphere of the womb. To comfort a cranky baby, try running a vacuum cleaner or a radio station that plays only static.

Swaddling

Another way to try to recreate the feel of the womb is through a tight swaddle. Swaddle your baby in a light blanket or use a special swaddling blanket made for this purpose.

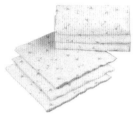

NEVER SHAKE YOUR BABY

It can be frustrating, exhausting, and even maddening dealing with a baby who cries for hours on end, while you're powerless to help. But never shake your infant. Shaking a baby can cause serious brain damage or even death. Instead, take a break if you're overwhelmed. Call a family member or babysitter to relieve you, or walk out of the room for a few minutes and breathe. And remember that this is temporary—colic generally subsides within a few months.

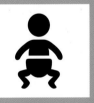

❧ CONGESTION ❧

A stuffy nose can make for a miserable day—and a worse night, if difficulty breathing keeps you awake. Congestion occurs when inflamed blood vessels cause tissues lining the nose to swell. In an attempt to flush out the source of the irritation, these tissues produce extra mucus. Sometimes this leads to a runny nose, and, if mucus continues into the throat, a postnasal drip. Congestion is often caused by colds, allergies, and sinus infections. Many people rely on over-the-counter decongestants and nasal sprays, while allergy sufferers may use antihistamines to deal with their congestion. For natural alternatives to these medications, try the following approaches.

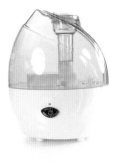

Steam

Thinning the mucus will help move it out of your nose and sinuses, offering some relief from congestion. Try using a vaporizer or humidifier in your bedroom. If you don't have one of these, you can also sit in the bathroom while the shower is running (make sure the steam isn't too hot, to avoid burns). The humidity will add moisture to the air, and make for easier breathing.

WHEN CONGESTION DOESN'T GO AWAY

If you've had a stuffy nose or sinus pressure for more than a week, call your doctor. This may be a sign that an infection has developed, requiring medical attention (and possibly antibiotics).

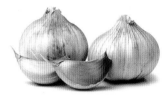

Garlic

For congestion related to a cold, consider garlic. With its antibacterial and antifungal properties, garlic has been found to be useful against colds and their symptoms. You can eat a few cloves of raw garlic, or, if you prefer, place the cloves in a pot of water, heat it, and inhale the steam from a safe distance.

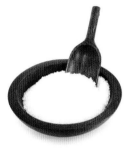

Salt Water

Salt water can keep your nasal passages moist while flushing out mucus, allergens, and other irritants. Nasal irrigators are available in stores, or you can use a neti pot or a syringe to irrigate your nasal passages with salt water. Boil water and let it cool before adding the salt.

Eucalyptus Oil

Eucalyptus oil helps to break up phlegm, easing congestion. Add a few drops of eucalyptus oil to a steaming bowl of water; then drape a towel around your head and the bowl, and inhale the steam (from a safe distance, again to avoid burns) for five to ten minutes.

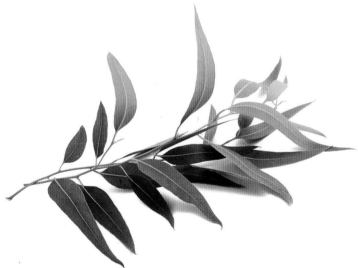

❧ CONJUNCTIVITIS ☙

Better known as "pink eye," conjunctivitis is an inflammation of the clear tissue lining the inside of the eyelid and covering the white part of the eye. Conjunctivitis can occur in one or both eyes, and symptoms may include a "gritty" feeling, redness and itchiness, excessive tearing, discharge that forms a crust over one or both eyes, pink discoloration in the white of the eye, and swollen eyelids. Pink eye may be caused by bacteria, a virus, or allergens, and sometimes accompanies a cold. Bacterial conjunctivitis generally needs to be treated with antibiotics, which typically clear up pink eye within a few days. Viral conjunctivitis needs to run its course, which unfortunately can take weeks. However, certain home remedies can ease the discomfort and speed the healing of pink eye.

WARNING

Both viral and bacterial conjunctivitis are highly contagious. If you think you or your child has conjunctivitis, it's important to see a doctor and take proper precautions to avoid spreading this illness.

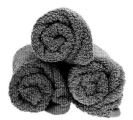

Cool Compress

While it won't clear up your pink eye any faster, a cool compress can soothe the itching and burning of conjunctivitis. Apply the compress directly to your closed eye. If you find it gives you greater relief, use a warm compress instead.

Salt Water

A saline solution can ease the symptoms of pink eye. Add ½–1 teaspoon of salt to 1 cup of water. Boil the mixture and allow to cool completely. Use a sterile dropper to rinse the eye with the solution several times a day.

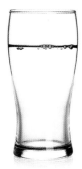

ALLERGIC CONJUNCTIVITIS

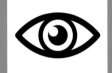

Sometimes allergies can lead to pink eye. In such cases, the first step is the same as with any allergy symptom—try to eliminate the allergen from your environment. If this doesn't work, your doctor may prescribe antihistamines or non-steroidal anti-inflammatory drugs. Managing allergy-related pink eye is similar to managing other allergy symptoms. Talk to your doctor about the best way to keep this symptom under control.

Honey

Used medicinally since ancient times, honey has antibacterial and antiviral properties, and can reduce pain and inflammation. Boil water and let it cool until it's warm. Dissolve ¼ teaspoon raw honey in one ¼ water. Use a sterile dropper to apply a couple of drops to the affected eye every few hours until symptoms subside.

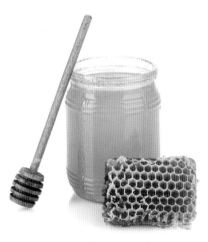

❧ CONSTIPATION ❧

Whether or not we like to admit it, everyone experiences constipation at points. Signs of constipation include having fewer than three bowel movements a week, straining during bowel movements, hard or small stools, a feeling of incomplete bowel movement, and rectal bleeding from hard stools. Many factors can cause constipation, including lack of fiber and water in the diet, too much dairy, lack of exercise, stress, and pregnancy. While there are a few serious conditions that cause constipation, for most people, a few diet and lifestyle changes can get things moving.

Fiber

Fiber is material made by plants that is unable to be digested by our bodies. As fiber passes through the digestive tract, it binds to water, softening and adding volume to stools—making them pass more easily through the intestines. The general recommended amount of fiber is 14 grams per 1,000 calories consumed. The World Health Organization recommends five servings a day of fruits and vegetables to ensure adequate intake of dietary fiber. Other sources of dietary fiber include whole grains, beans, and nuts. Add fiber slowly, to avoid bloating and gas.

Lemon

The citric acid in lemons can stimulate the digestive system and help to expel undigested material lingering in the colon's walls. Squeeze the juice of a lemon into a glass of warm water and enjoy a relaxing drink.

> ## PRUNES: NATURES LAXATIVE
>
> If you're looking to add fiber to your diet, consider prunes. This wonder-fruit contains sorbitol, which acts as a natural laxative in the body, and is high in dietary fiber. In fact, 1 cup of prunes contains 12 grams of fiber—almost the entire recommended amount per 1,000 calories you eat!

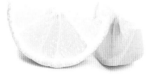

GET MOVING!

Exercise isn't just for building muscle and losing fat. It also eases constipation, by helping to move food through your large intestine. Walking is especially beneficial for pregnant women suffering from constipation. Try a twenty to thirty minute daily walk to improve your overall health—including your digestion.

Water

Water softens the stool and makes intestines smooth and flexible, for easier passage of waste. If the large intestine doesn't have enough water, it'll seek it out elsewhere—like in your stools, making them hard and painful. To avoid this problem, drink plenty of water—conventionally eight 8-ounce glasses a day for healthy people (which may vary depending on weight, age, and other factors). And avoid alcohol, which can dehydrate your body.

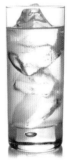

Magnesium

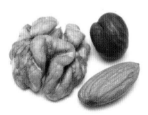

Magnesium, an active ingredient in many over-the-counter laxative medicines, relieves constipation by relaxing muscles in the walls of the intestines. You can find this mineral in foods such as dark leafy greens, nuts, and beans. Or, you can take a magnesium supplement, 200 milligrams a day.

❧ COUGHS ❧

While it may sound terrible, a cough is simply your body's way of clearing irritants and mucus out of the lungs and airways. Coughs can be caused by a variety of factors, from dust in the air to the common cold to more serious conditions such as bronchitis or pneumonia. Doctors refer to two types of cough: *productive*, in which you cough up phlegm or mucus; and *nonproductive*, or a dry cough. A cough that brings up greenish, yellow phlegm may be a sign of an infection, which needs to be treated by a doctor. Many people relieve their coughs with over-the-counter expectorants, which thin the mucus, and suppressants, which suppress the cough reflex. For natural alternatives to relieve your cough, try one of these simple remedies from your kitchen.

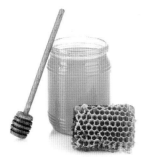

Honey

To suppress a dry, hacking cough, try a little bit of honey, which soothes and coats irritated mucus membranes. Take 1 tablespoon of organic, raw honey several times a day.

Steam

Steam can loosen mucus phlegm, allowing you to more easily cough it up. You can sit in the bathroom while running a warm shower, or boil enough water to fill a bowl, allow it to cool slightly, and breathe in the steam while holding a towel over your head and the bowl (from a safe distance, so you don't burn yourself). For added antibacterial benefits, add a few drops of tea tree oil.

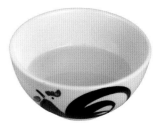

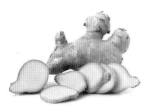

Ginger

A natural antihistamine and decongestant, ginger can treat many cold and flu symptoms, including coughs. To make ginger tea, combine twelve slices of ginger with 3 cups of water in a pot and simmer for twenty minutes. Remove from heat and strain; add a tablespoon of honey for extra relief.

WHEN A COUGH IS SERIOUS

Contact your doctor if your cough is accompanied by any of the following:

- Fever

- Shortness of breath

- Chest pain

- Wheezing

- Yellow-greenish phlegm

Also contact your child's pediatrician if the cough resembles "barking," as this is often a characteristic sign of croup.

Thyme

Thyme reduces inflammation, opens the airways, and relaxes the muscles of the bronchi and trachea. Make thyme tea by mixing 2 teaspoons crushed thyme leaves in 1 cup boiling water. Cover and steep for ten minutes before straining.

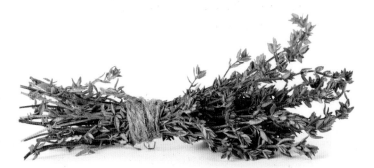

⤙ CUTS AND ABRASIONS ⤙

Whether your child fell off his bike and onto the pavement, or you got a little too aggressive chopping the vegetables, the resulting cut or abrasion can be painful and should be dealt with immediately. A cut can cause bleeding and, if bacteria enter the wound, may lead to infection. Abrasions are often less serious, tending to affect the outermost layer of skin. Abrasions occur when your skin moves against a rough surface, leading to a rubbing away of the topmost layers of skin—something parents commonly see when their kids play soccer, for example. No matter what kind of wound you or your child has, your priority—once you've stopped the bleeding, of course—is to promote healing and prevent infection or scarring.

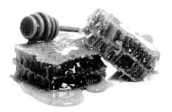

Honey

Honey has antibacterial and pain-relieving properties, and may help prevent scarring. Clean the cut or abrasion with soap and water, and then apply a thin layer of honey and a bandage.

Tea Tree Oil

A natural antiseptic, tea tree oil fights bacteria and aids in healing. Create a mixture of 50 percent tea tree oil and 50 percent olive oil, and apply the combination directly to the wound.

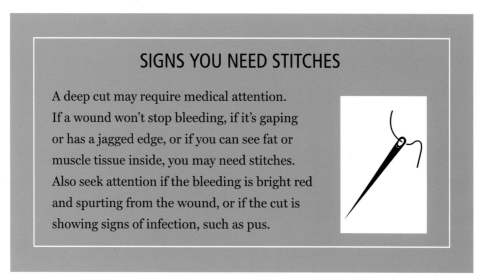

SIGNS YOU NEED STITCHES

A deep cut may require medical attention. If a wound won't stop bleeding, if it's gaping or has a jagged edge, or if you can see fat or muscle tissue inside, you may need stitches. Also seek attention if the bleeding is bright red and spurting from the wound, or if the cut is showing signs of infection, such as pus.

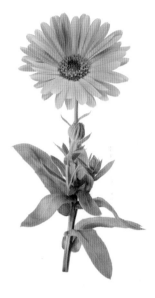

Calendula

Also known as pot marigold or garden marigold, *calendula officinalis* has antimicrobial properties and anti-inflammatory properties, making it a useful treatment for cuts and abrasions. Apply the crushed plant directly to the wound; or dilute calendula tincture with water, soak a cotton ball in the mixture, and secure it on the wound with a bandage.

WARNING

Do not ingest or use calendula topically if you are pregnant or breastfeeding, or if you are allergic to ragweed, marigolds, or other related plants. Talk to your doctor about your allergies before taking calendula.

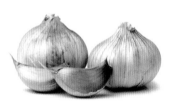

Garlic

Another natural bacteria-fighter from your kitchen, garlic contains allicin, an antimicrobial agent that protects against infection. Tape a clove of garlic directly to a cut or scrape; however, as garlic is irritating to the skin, do not leave on for more than twenty to twenty-five minutes.

Onion

Like garlic, onions also contain the antimicrobial agent allicin. Fortunately, onions are less irritating to the skin. Apply some crushed onion to the area for thirty minutes or so, three times a day.

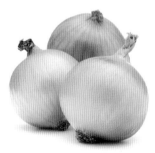

DANDRUFF

Talk about embarrassing: You put on your best black dress or jacket, head out to a special event, and later discover that your shoulders are covered in white flakes. Dandruff occurs when your scalp sheds dead skin cells. While it's normal to shed a certain amount of skin cells, for some people, the condition is more severe and can be accompanied by itching and scales on the scalp. Causes of dandruff include dry skin, especially in dry, winter weather; failure to shampoo enough, causing a buildup of skin cells from your scalp; a yeast-like fungus that can irritate the scalp; and skin conditions such as eczema. While medicated, over-the-counter shampoos can help treat dandruff, various natural remedies can stop the flakes as well.

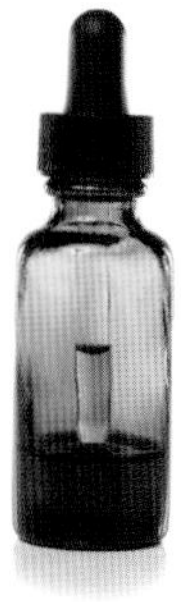

Tea Tree Oil

Tea tree oil has antifungal properties and can penetrate and unclog hair follicles, getting to the root of those annoying flakes. Many shampoos contain tree oil, or you can mix a few drops of tea tree oil with a few drops of olive oil, wet your hair, and massage the mixture onto your scalp with your fingertips. Leave on for one hour before washing your hair with shampoo and conditioner.

Olive Oil

While too much oil on the scalp can trigger dandruff, the right amount can moisturize the skin, and soften and release scales that would otherwise flake into dandruff so you can wash them away. Warm a few ounces of olive oil on the stove (not hot enough to burn your scalp!), wet your hair, and massage the oil directly onto your scalp. Leave on for half an hour and then rinse. For severe cases, after massaging the oil into your scalp, cover it with a shower cap and leave on overnight, rinsing in the morning with a dandruff shampoo.

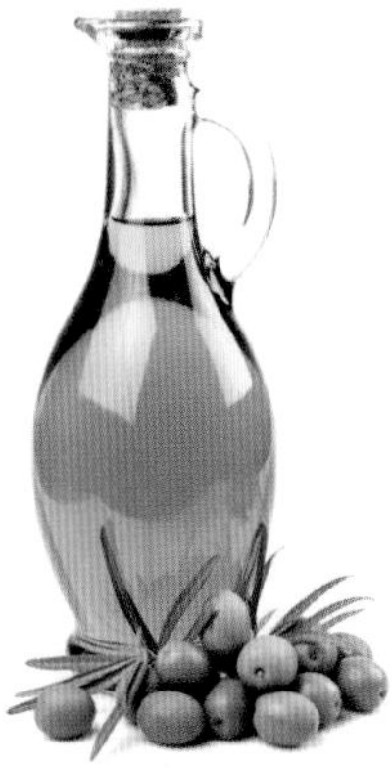

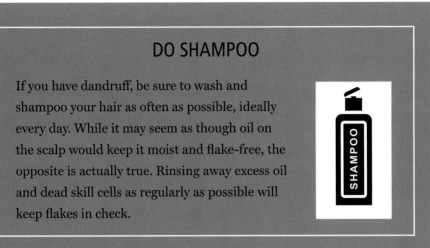

DO SHAMPOO

If you have dandruff, be sure to wash and shampoo your hair as often as possible, ideally every day. While it may seem as though oil on the scalp would keep it moist and flake-free, the opposite is actually true. Rinsing away excess oil and dead skill cells as regularly as possible will keep flakes in check.

Vinegar

To eliminate dead skin cells that cause dandruff, rinse your hair with vinegar. Vinegar also kills fungus, another potential source of dandruff. Mix ½ cup white vinegar or apple cider vinegar with ½ cup warm water, and gently rub the mixture into your hair before rinsing with water.

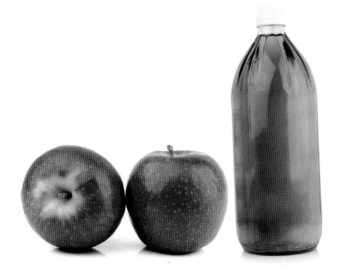

❧ DIAPER RASH ❦

Oh, baby! Few things upset a new parent like taking off baby's diaper, only to find red, irritated skin underneath. Diaper rash is often caused by moisture on baby's skin, which may occur if the diaper isn't changed quickly enough, or if the child has particularly sensitive skin. Some babies are allergic or sensitive to chemicals present in different diapers. Others may be reacting to new foods that change the frequency or composition of their stools. And, in some cases, the warm, moist area under the diaper attracts yeast and bacteria, leading to an infection and rash. No matter what the cause, a diaper rash can leave your baby irritated and uncomfortable. Fortunately, there are various remedies to ease baby's pain.

Oatmeal

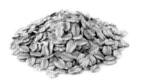

Skin-soothing, healing oatmeal is also great to add to baby's bath. Place ⅓ cup oatmeal in a blender, and blend until it forms a fine powder. Sprinkle the oatmeal in the bath and stir with your hands. Allow your child to soak in the tub for ten to fifteen minutes.

Coconut Oil

Coconut oil soothes the skin and has antifungal properties that help to fight the yeast responsible for some rashes. It also forms a barrier between baby's bottom and feces and urine. After each diaper change, wash baby's bottom with water and allow to dry. Apply a thin layer of coconut oil with your fingertips and cover with a clean diaper.

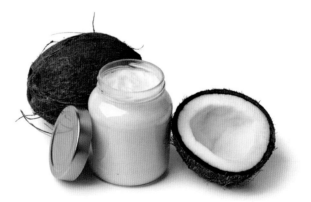

LOSE THOSE WIPES

Sometimes, alcohol or chemicals in commercial diaper wipes can irritate a baby's bottom and cause diaper rash. If your baby is prone to diaper rash, try using a spray bottle of warm water to rinse his or her bottom during a diaper change. For wiping up baby after a bowel movement, you can use a soft cloth soaked in warm water and soap.

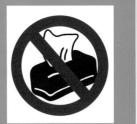

Baking Soda

Baking soda has antibacterial and antifungal properties, and can soothe irritated skin. Add 2 tablespoons of baking soda to baby's bathwater and bathe your child as usual.

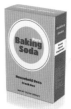

WARNING

If your baby's umbilical cord has not yet fallen off, consult your doctor before giving baby a bath, as many doctors recommend sponge baths only during this time. And never, ever leave an infant unsupervised in the tub.

❧ DIARRHEA ❧

Diarrhea refers to watery, loose bowel movements. It's often caused by a virus and referred to as the "stomach flu"; however, other causes include bacterial infection, food allergies, side effects from medications, and more chronic conditions like irritable bowel syndrome (see page 128). In addition to loose stools, diarrhea can cause bloating, abdominal cramps, nausea, and a feeling of having to go—right *now!* Over-the-counter medications exist to treat diarrhea, or you can let it run its course, which may take two to three days. However, to soothe the symptoms and speed recovery naturally, try one of these simple approaches.

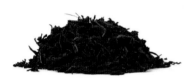

Black Tea

The tannins in tea help to reduce intestinal inflammation, and black tea can help to rehydrate you after a bout of diarrhea. Let the tea steep for fifteen minutes and drink as necessary to ease symptoms.

Blackberries

Like black tea, blackberries also contain astringent tannins that can ease the symptoms of diarrhea. You can buy blackberry tea or make your own by boiling 1 to 2 tablespoons of blackberries in 1½ cups water for ten minutes and then straining. Or, you can pour 1 cup of boiling water over 2 teaspoons of dried blackberry leaves. Steep for ten minutes and then strain.

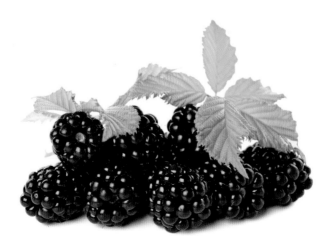

Probiotics

If bacteria are to blame for your digestive troubles, probiotics can repopulate the digestive tract with "good" bacteria. Look for probiotic supplements, or add probiotic-containing foods such as kefir or yogurt (containing "live active cultures") to your diet. Also add probiotics to your diet when taking antibiotics, to maintain the balance of bacteria in your digestive system.

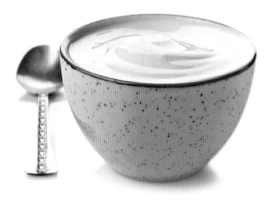

THE BRAT DIET

After diarrhea, it's often a good idea to stick to bland, binding foods to help ease your way back to normal digestion. BRAT is an acronym for bananas, rice, applesauce, and toast. These foods are low-fiber, making for firmer stools; in addition, the potassium in bananas can help to replace lost nutrients. Follow this diet for the first twenty-four to forty-eight hours after diarrhea, and then begin to re-introduce other foods into your meals.

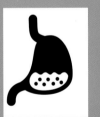

❧ DRY MOUTH ❧

Also known as xerostomia, dry mouth occurs when you don't produce enough saliva to moisten your mouth and digest food. Symptoms can range from a sticky feeling in your mouth to bad breath, excessive thirst, and even problems chewing and swallowing. Dry mouth can be caused by dehydration, smoking, medical conditions, or as a side effect of certain drugs, such as antihistamines and drugs used to treat depression and anxiety. Dry mouth also puts you at risk of developing gum disease and tooth decay. While a doctor may prescribe medication, certain kitchen cures can relieve symptoms and restore moisture to your dry mouth.

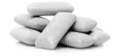

Sugarless Candy and Gum

To stimulate saliva production, suck on sugarless candy or gum. Sugarless gums containing xylitol also battle bacteria, which can contribute to bad breath, cavities, and other oral health problems. To further stimulate saliva flow, go for a citrus-flavored candy.

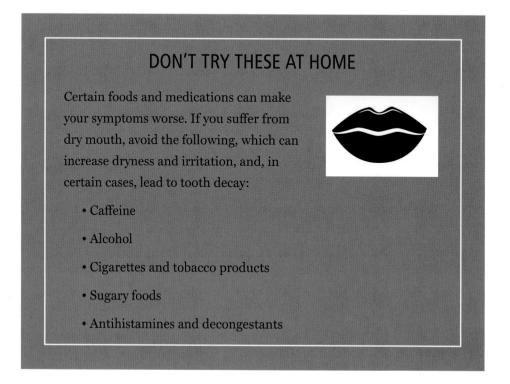

DON'T TRY THESE AT HOME

Certain foods and medications can make your symptoms worse. If you suffer from dry mouth, avoid the following, which can increase dryness and irritation, and, in certain cases, lead to tooth decay:

- Caffeine

- Alcohol

- Cigarettes and tobacco products

- Sugary foods

- Antihistamines and decongestants

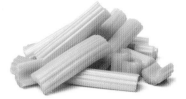

Celery

Foods with high water content such as celery, cucumbers, or watermelon can moisturize the mouth and stimulate the salivary glands. Munch on celery whenever your mouth is dry—and when you want a nutritious snack!

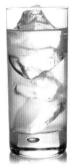

Water

Drinking water can keep your mouth lubricated and counter the many effects of dry mouth. Conventional guidelines suggest that healthy people should drink at least eight 8-ounce glasses a day, although these guidelines may vary depending on your weight, age, and activity level. When you go to the gym, be sure to bring a water bottle and hydrate throughout your workout.

Cayenne Pepper

Red pepper doesn't just stimulate your tear ducts and sweat glands, it also activates your salivary glands as well. Sprinkle it on your food or add some mouth-watering salsa to your dinner plate.

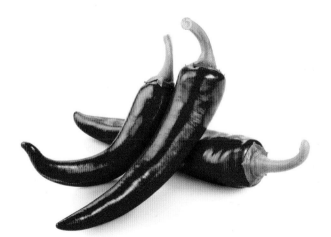

❧ DRY SKIN ❧

The old adage says, "Love the skin you're in." But that can be hard to do when your skin is tight, dry, and itchy. Dry skin is often caused by external factors, such as winter weather, heating systems that reduce humidity and dry the skin, and hot showers combined with moisture-stripping soaps. People with certain medical conditions such as eczema may also experience dry skin. While drugstores may be filled with expensive moisturizers, the remedies below can help you feel comfortable in your own skin—without spending a fortune.

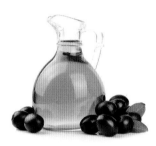

Olive Oil

Olive oil moisturizes dry skin, and has antioxidants to help protect the skin from the damaging effects of the sun. Apply the olive oil directly to your dry skin for a boost of moisture. Be careful, however, about using olive oil on your face if you're prone to breakouts. In that case, consider a beauty product that contains olive oil but is noncomedogenic, meaning it won't block your pores.

Coconut Oil

Is there anything coconut oil can't do? It has antifungal and antimicrobial properties—and it's a natural moisturizer. In fact, a 2013 study published in the *International Journal of Dermatology* found that virgin coconut oil decreased water loss in the skin of patients with atopic dermatitis, a condition that prevents the skin from retaining moisture. Apply topically once or twice a day and after bathing.

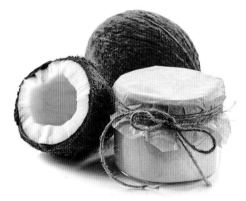

Grapeseed Oil

High in vitamin C, grapeseed oil—which comes from the seeds of pressed grapes—can brighten and moisturize the skin. And, since grapeseed oil is fairly light, it is easily absorbed into the skin without leaving an oily residue. Use it as you would a regular moisturizer.

Aloe Vera

Aloe vera gel moisturizes dry skin and softens dead skin cells, making them easier to remove. To use the gel as a moisturizer, split open a leaf from a plant, scoop out the gel, and apply it directly to the affected area.

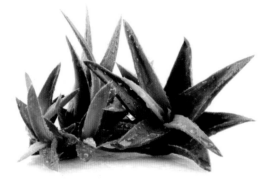

WASH WISELY

If you suffer from dry skin, limit the amount of time you spend in the shower or tub. Hot water and lengthy showers can strip oil from your skin. Use warm water, and try to spend ten minutes or less bathing. If your skin is really dry, try bathing a few times a week instead of every day.

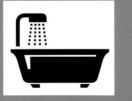

❧ EARACHE ❧

Common among children, earaches can be quite painful and lead to missed days of school and sleepless nights. Earaches are caused by many factors, including the common cold, a sinus infection, or an infection of the middle ear. Commonly, when we experience ear pain, it's because the Eustachian tubes—the passageways from the back of the throat to the middle ear—are clogged with mucus. As fluid builds up there, a bacterial or viral infection can develop, characterized by sharp pain, loss of appetite, fever, and other symptoms. While earaches caused by colds often go away on their own, over-the-counter pain medications can ease the discomfort of an earache—or, you can try one of the natural remedies below.

WARNING

Because an earache can lead to an infection, especially in children, it's important to see a doctor if the earache lasts longer than a week, is excessively painful, or is accompanied by a fever. If you have any symptoms of a ruptured eardrum—sudden sharp pain that gradually ceases, discharge from the ear, dizziness, or any changes in your hearing—see a doctor immediately and seek his or her medical opinion before trying any home or over-the-counter remedies.

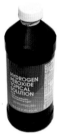

Hydrogen Peroxide

Hydrogen peroxide can dislodge debris, while calming inflammation and disinfecting. Using a bulb syringe or a soaked cotton ball, apply 3–5 drops of hydrogen peroxide into the affected ear canal. Lie with the painful ear facing up; after ten minutes, turn your head and slowly let the peroxide drain from your ear.

Olive Oil

Warm olive oil in the ear canal can soothe an inflamed eardrum. Using a dropper, apply a few drops in the ear canal and lie with the affected ear facing up few several minutes, so that the olive oil can reach the eardrum.

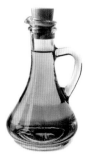

Heat

To dull the pain of an earache, apply warmth, in the form of a wet washcloth, warm towel from the clothes dryer, or a heating pad set on low. Parents should never leave a child unsupervised around hot objects.

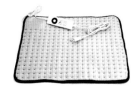

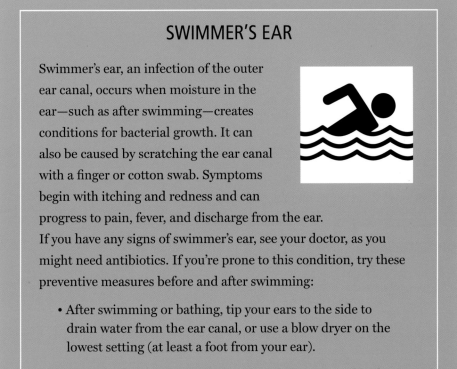

SWIMMER'S EAR

Swimmer's ear, an infection of the outer ear canal, occurs when moisture in the ear—such as after swimming—creates conditions for bacterial growth. It can also be caused by scratching the ear canal with a finger or cotton swab. Symptoms begin with itching and redness and can progress to pain, fever, and discharge from the ear.

If you have any signs of swimmer's ear, see your doctor, as you might need antibiotics. If you're prone to this condition, try these preventive measures before and after swimming:

- After swimming or bathing, tip your ears to the side to drain water from the ear canal, or use a blow dryer on the lowest setting (at least a foot from your ear).

- Dab petroleum jelly inside the edge of your ear to absorb moisture.

- Mix one part rubbing alcohol with one part white vinegar. Pour a teaspoon into each ear and then tip your head to drain it out. This drying agent can also ward off bacteria and fungi.

With a little effort, you can reduce your risk of swimmer's ear—and stop avoiding the pool.

⁓ ECZEMA ⁓

Eczema causes red, itchy inflammation of the skin. Atopic dermatitis, a common form of eczema, generally affects children and can continue periodically throughout adulthood. Other symptoms may include dry, scaly skin and crusty patches. Doctors aren't exactly sure what causes eczema, but one theory is that's an overreaction of the immune system to an allergen in the environment. Doctors generally recommend controlling the itching and dryness of eczema with lotions and products that lubricate the skin, or with prescription creams containing corticosteroids or other medications. To get that eczema itch under control, you could also try one of the natural remedies on the next page.

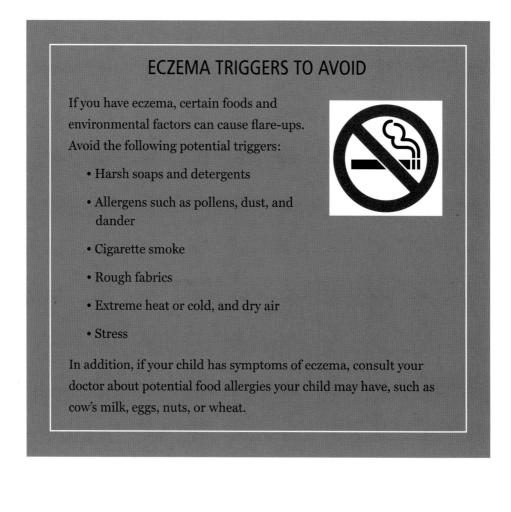

ECZEMA TRIGGERS TO AVOID

If you have eczema, certain foods and environmental factors can cause flare-ups. Avoid the following potential triggers:

- Harsh soaps and detergents

- Allergens such as pollens, dust, and dander

- Cigarette smoke

- Rough fabrics

- Extreme heat or cold, and dry air

- Stress

In addition, if your child has symptoms of eczema, consult your doctor about potential food allergies your child may have, such as cow's milk, eggs, nuts, or wheat.

Oatmeal

Colloidal, or finely ground, oatmeal is an ingredient in various over-the-counter eczema creams. To soothe itchy skin, add one of these products to your bath—or, make your own colloidal oatmeal by placing oatmeal in a blender, and blending until it forms a fine powder. (Use 2 cups for adults and 1 cup for children.) Sprinkle the oatmeal in lukewarm bathwater and stir with your hands. Make sure the water isn't too hot, and don't soak for more than ten minutes, as this may make the eczema worse. Moisturize your skin within a few minutes of leaving the tub.

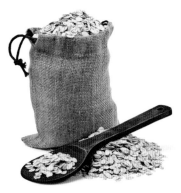

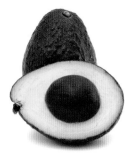

Avocado

Rich in healthy fats and vitamins A, D, and E, avocados can help reduce skin inflammation and relieve eczema symptoms. Add avocados to your meals to treat eczema from the inside out, and apply mashed avocados or avocado oil topically to red, itchy areas to soothe them.

Aloe Vera

With its moisturizing, anti-inflammatory, and antimicrobial properties, aloe vera can relieve the inflammation and itchiness of eczema. Apply fresh gel from an aloe vera plant directly to the affected area. The plant is preferable to over-the-counter gels, which may contain alcohol that can dry the skin.

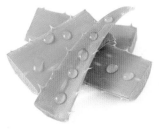

➤ EYE IRRITATION AND EYESTRAIN ➤

Everyone appreciates eye contact—unless it's with dust, dry air, or allergens, of course. Red, itchy, dry eyes caused by an irritant can be painful and unattractive. Similarly, eyestrain caused by overuse—such as sitting in front of a computer for hours on end—can also cause problems, such as blurred vision, burning or itchy eyes, and headaches. Fortunately, there are some simple lifestyle changes and home remedies available to ease irritation and eyestrain, so you can see the world clearly (and comfortably) once more.

WARNING

Consult a doctor if you experience eye pain, dizziness, continued headaches, sensitivity to light, double or change of vision, or if home treatments fail to relieve the irritation.

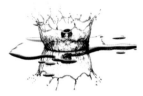

Cool Water

To ease inflammation and soothe strained eyes, run a washcloth under cool water and then place it over your closed eyes. Leave the washcloth in place until your eyes start to feel better.

Cucumbers

A common remedy for puffy, irritated eyes, cucumbers contain antioxidants and flavonoids that are thought to reduce irritation. Thinly slice a cucumber, and then refrigerate the slices for fifteen minutes. Place one slice on each closed eye and leave on for four to five minutes.

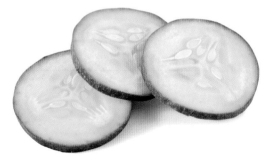

EYE-FRIENDLY COMPUTER WORK

If you're experiencing eyestrain you may have your computer to blame. Nonstop staring at a brightly lit, flat screen can make anyone's eyes tired. To protect your eyes while at the computer, try these tips:

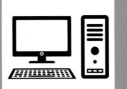

- **Keep your distance.** Position the monitor twenty to forty inches from you, and make sure the top of the screen is eye level or slightly lower, so that you're looking down at it.

- **Lower the lighting.** The screen's bright light promotes eyestrain, so dim the screen to a comfortable level and adjust the contrast so you can easily read the letters on the screen.

- **Avoid glare.** Try to position your computer so that light sources above and behind you don't cause glare on the screen. Close the blinds or shades if you can.

And, most importantly, remember to give your eyes a break. Walk away from your screen every couple of hours, and for every twenty minutes of computer work, look at an object twenty feet away for at least twenty seconds. Your eyes will thank you.

Potatoes

Similar to cumbers, vitamin C-rich potato slices can relieve itchy, irritated eyes. Refrigerate slices of raw potato for thirty minutes, and then place a slice on each closed eye.

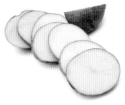

❧ FATIGUE ❧

Imagine all the things you could get done if you had more energy—landscaping the yard, playing more with the kids, going on that long-postponed hiking trip. The exhaustion and low energy of fatigue can have many causes, including lack of sleep, overactivity, certain medications, drinking alcohol or caffeine, stress, anxiety, and depression. While constant exhaustion may be a sign of an underlying medical condition, most cases of fatigue are temporary. With a few basic lifestyle changes and home remedies, you can regain the energy you need to conquer the world—or at least make it through the workday.

LIFESTYLE MATTERS

One of the best ways to combat fatigue and give yourself an energy boost is by making certain lifestyle changes:

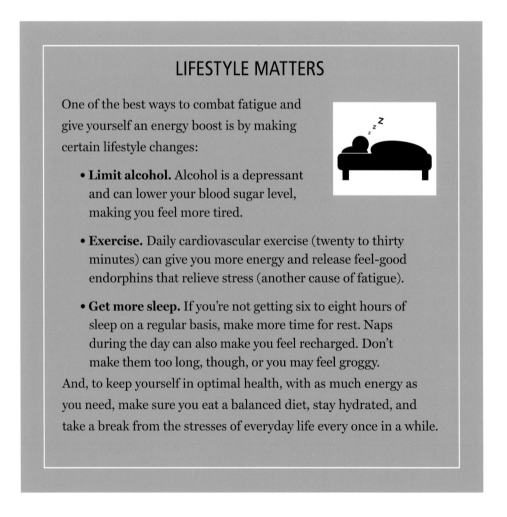

- **Limit alcohol.** Alcohol is a depressant and can lower your blood sugar level, making you feel more tired.

- **Exercise.** Daily cardiovascular exercise (twenty to thirty minutes) can give you more energy and release feel-good endorphins that relieve stress (another cause of fatigue).

- **Get more sleep.** If you're not getting six to eight hours of sleep on a regular basis, make more time for rest. Naps during the day can also make you feel recharged. Don't make them too long, though, or you may feel groggy.

And, to keep yourself in optimal health, with as much energy as you need, make sure you eat a balanced diet, stay hydrated, and take a break from the stresses of everyday life every once in a while.

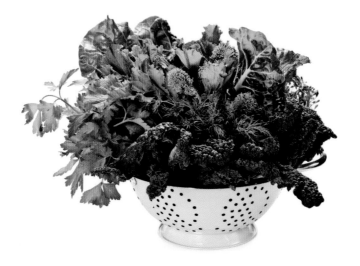

Magnesium

Your body uses magnesium in hundreds of reactions, a good portion of which provide you with energy. Low levels of magnesium can lead to fewer available red blood cells and lower energy. Magnesium is present in foods such as dark leafy greens, nuts, and beans. Or, look for a magnesium supplement, 200 milligrams a day.

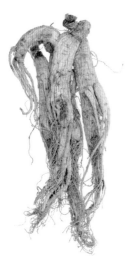

Ginseng

Ginseng has long been known to naturally provide energy. In a 2010 study at the Mayo Clinic, more than twice as many cancer patients taking ginseng reported less fatigue and increased energy compared with those given the placebo. You can find ginseng supplements at health food stores. Take two 100-milligram capsules a day, or follow the dosage on the label.

❧ FEVER ❧

Chills. Aching muscles. Loss of appetite. The signs of a fever are easy to identify, even before the thermometer confirms the diagnosis. If you or your child has a fever, take heart. A fever is merely a sign that your body is working to fight off an infection, by raising your body temperature so it's less hospitable to bacteria and viruses. For adults, a fever begins when the thermometer goes above the "normal" 98.6°F, although everyone's average temperature is slightly different, so your fever point may vary. According to the American Academy of Pediatrics (AAP), for kids, most pediatricians consider a temperature above 100.4°F to be a sign of a fever. While a fever may be miserable, it generally subsides within a few days. To deal with the aches and pains of a fever, try these home remedies.

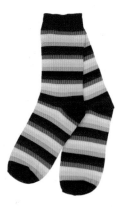

Socks

Yes, you read that right. To navigate the heat of a fever away from your head and to your feet, try soaking a pair of socks in egg whites and placing them on your feet until they dry out. Use two to three egg whites for children and five for adults. In lieu of eggs, you can also use warm lemon juice or apple cider vinegar.

Willow Bark Tea

People have been using willow bark to relieve fever and inflammation since the days of Hippocrates (400 BCE). It contains salicin, a chemical similar to aspirin. To make tea from the dried herb, boil 1–2 teaspoons of dried bark in 8 ounces of water; simmer for ten to fifteen minutes and let it steep for half an hour.

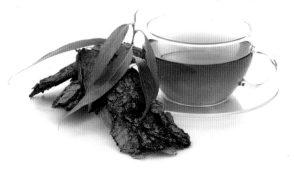

HOW HIGH IS TOO HIGH?

Call a doctor immediately if your temperature is 103°F or higher, if you have a fever higher than 101°F that lasts for more than three days, or if you're experiencing a stiff neck, trouble breathing, or vomiting. For infants under 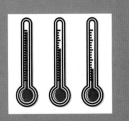 three months, call your pediatrician at any sign of a fever. For children older than three months, the AAP advises calling the doctor if:

- Fever rises above 104°F

- Fever lasts longer than twenty-four hours in a child younger than two years

- Fever lasts longer than three days in a child who's two or older

- Fever is accompanied by other symptoms such as ear pain, vomiting, or a seizure

If you're unsure, trust your gut: call your child's doctor if your child is unusually fussy, tired, or just isn't acting like himself.

Cayenne Pepper

If you can muster up an appetite, add some cayenne pepper to your food. The capsaicin in these peppers will get your blood flowing and help you sweat out that fever.

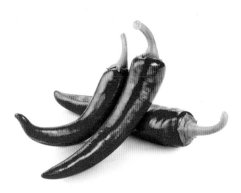

❧ FLATULENCE ❧

Flatulence may be a funny subject to some, but if you find yourself excessively passing gas, you're probably not laughing. Flatulence refers to having too much gas or air in the digestive system. This can occur from swallowing air, consuming certain foods and beverages, or as a side effect of medications or hormonal shifts. Passing gas is a normal bodily function; in fact, the UK's National Health Service estimates that people pass gas on average fifteen times a day. However, if excessive flatulence is causing you discomfort or embarrassment, there are natural ways to address this awkward problem.

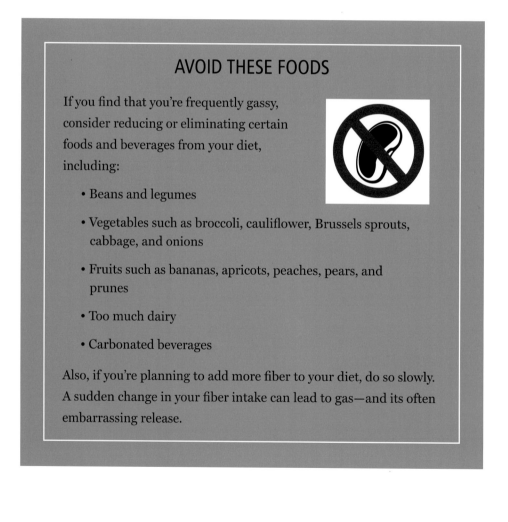

AVOID THESE FOODS

If you find that you're frequently gassy, consider reducing or eliminating certain foods and beverages from your diet, including:

- Beans and legumes

- Vegetables such as broccoli, cauliflower, Brussels sprouts, cabbage, and onions

- Fruits such as bananas, apricots, peaches, pears, and prunes

- Too much dairy

- Carbonated beverages

Also, if you're planning to add more fiber to your diet, do so slowly. A sudden change in your fiber intake can lead to gas—and its often embarrassing release.

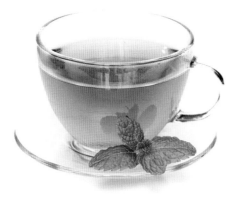

Peppermint Tea

Peppermint can reduce gas and relieve spasms in the gastrointestinal tract, aiding digestion. Add dried peppermint leaves to 1 cup of boiled water and steep for five to ten minutes. Strain and drink 1–2 cups a day.

Fennel Seeds

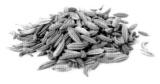

Fennel, a plant indigenous to the Mediterranean region, has long been used to treat gas. It's a natural carminative, meaning it either prevents the formation of gas or eases its release, so it doesn't build up in your digestive system. Fennel is also rich in minerals and antioxidants that ease digestion. You can chew on the seeds or add them to a meal. Or, boil a few seeds in water for five minutes, strain, and allow the liquid to cool before drinking.

Caraway Seeds

Like fennel seeds, caraway seeds are also carminatives, and reduce gas. Add them to your food, or indulge in caraway-seed crackers as a snack.

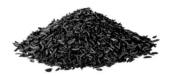

❧ FOOD POISONING ❧

You are what you eat—and if your food's contaminated with bacteria, viruses, or toxins, chances are you're about to be sick. Contamination can occur at any point in a food's production or preparation, from when it's harvested on the farm to when it's stored in the supermarket or cooked in your kitchen. Symptoms of food poisoning may take hours or days to appear, and may include vomiting, nausea, diarrhea, abdominal cramping, and fever. While most cases of food poisoning generally clear up on their own, sometimes medical treatment is necessary. To ease the symptoms of food poisoning, try these natural, soothing remedies.

WARNING

Call the doctor if you are continuously vomiting and can't hold down liquids, have a fever higher than 101.5°F, there's blood in your vomit or diarrhea, you're dehydrated, or you're experiencing other symptoms such as blurry vision or difficulty breathing.

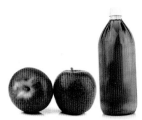

Apple Cider Vinegar

ACV has antibacterial and anti-inflammatory properties, as well as an alkaline effect on the body, that can ease digestive stress and symptoms of food poisoning. Mix 2 teaspoons ACV in 1cup warm water, and drink the mixture several times a day.

Basil

Certain cooking herbs, such as basil, have microbial properties that combat food-borne toxins. Add basil leaves to 3 tablespoons of plain yogurt (with "live cultures," or good bacteria) and eat this three to four times a day. Other herbs with these properties include thyme, rosemary, coriander, sage, and fennel.

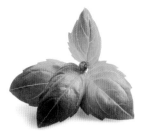

SAFETY FIRST

Handling food improperly can lead to contamination and sickness. To avoid exposing food to bacteria, follow these guidelines for storing and preparing food in your home:

- **Keep raw foods separate**. To prevent cross-contamination, keep raw meats and fish separate from other food items.

- **Keep it clean.** When handling raw foods and produce, wash your hands, utensils, cooking boards, and surfaces frequently with warm, soapy water.

- **Don't leave food out.** Defrost meat in the refrigerator and then cook it promptly. Place leftovers immediately in the refrigerator.

And, like your mother told you, "when in doubt, throw it out." If food smells or looks funny, is past its expiration date, or has been sitting out for a while, throw it away. It may feel wasteful, but you'll save yourself some grief in the long run.

Ginger Tea

Ginger has anti-inflammatory properties and can ease nausea and upset stomachs. You can make ginger tea by combining twelve slices of ginger with 3 cups of water in a pot and simmer for twenty minutes. Remove from heat and strain.

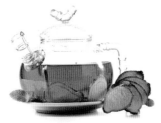

❧ FOOT ODOR ❧

Kids love making jokes about "smelly feet"—but if your shoes smell like a locker room, you may be dealing with a not-so-funny problem. According to the American Academy of Podiatric Practice Management, with around 3,000 glands per square inch, the feet and hands have more sweat glands than any other part of the body. When all that sweat is contained in tight-fitting shoes and socks, bacteria can thrive, producing an acid that, well, stinks. Fortunately, some simple home remedies can control the stink—and embarrassment—of foot odor.

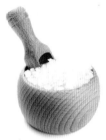

Salt Water

After walking around in sweaty socks and shoes all day, it's not surprising that the smell from the ground may be less than pleasant. Give your feet a relaxing, bacteria-fighting soak in a tub filled with 1 cup of salt for each quart of water. Let your feet air dry afterward.

Black Tea

The tannin in tea acts as a drying agent; in addition, the acid in tea is antibacterial and can close pores. Boil four tea bags in a quart of water for fifteen minutes. Add cool water and then soak your feet for at least twenty minutes.

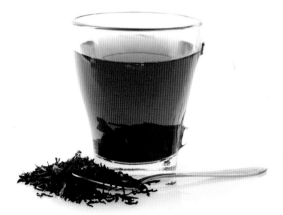

Raw Potatoes

You may feel silly placing potatoes on your feet, but this kitchen remedy can be a powerful tool in your odor-fighting arsenal. Chemicals in potatoes absorb toxins from the soles of your feet, helping to fight the foul smell. Place slices of raw organic potatoes in your socks and leave on overnight.

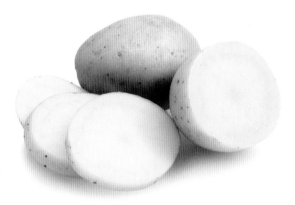

IF THE SHOE FITS . . .

The key to eliminating foot odor is to keep your feet dry, and therefore less hospitable to odor-causing bacteria. Wear clean socks to prevent sweat and bacteria from collecting in your shoes, and change your socks often. When possible, opt 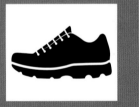 for footwear that allows your feet to breathe, such as sandals or open-toed shoes. Sprinkle some cornstarch in your shoes to absorb excess moisture. By taking care of your footwear, you can prevent odors and get back on your feet—without the embarrassment.

❧ GOUT ❧

A type of arthritis, gout is a condition that occurs when too much uric acid accumulates in the blood. As a result, sharp uric acid crystals build up in the joints, causing inflammation, pain, redness, and stiffness. Gout is most common in the joints of the big toe, but other joints can be affected as well. Your body produces uric acid when breaking down a substance called purines, found in high quantities in certain foods such as asparagus, liver, anchovies, and gravies. While uric acid normally passes through to the urine, if your body creates too much of it or your kidneys eliminate too little, gout can occur. Changing your diet may help manage gout, as can certain medications. Should you still find yourself experiencing the pain of this inflammatory condition, try these natural approaches for relief.

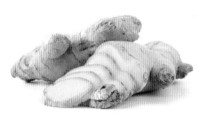

Ginger Root

Ginger root has anti-inflammatory properties to help relieve the pain of gout. Mix ½ teaspoon ginger root in 1 cup of boiling water, allow to cool, and drink. Or, add some water to ginger root to make a paste and apply directly to your toe or other affected area. Leave it on for half an hour before rinsing it off.

Cherries

A sweet way to prevent gout, cherries have been linked to fewer gout attacks and lower levels of uric acid. A study at Michigan State University showed that the anthocyanins that make cherries red also inhibit certain enzymes, in a way similar to how anti-inflammatory drugs reduce pain. According to the research, you'd have to eat the equivalent of twenty tart cherries to experience this effect.

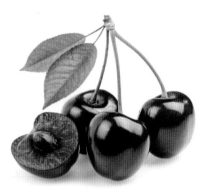

SAY NO TO ALCOHOL

If you're prone to attacks of gout, avoid drinking alcohol. Alcohol, especially beer, hinders your body's ability to remove uric acid. Water, on the other hand, helps eliminate uric acid—so drink up!

Coffee

Your morning cup of Joe may actually help relieve your gout. Scientists aren't sure why, but coffee has been associated with lower levels of uric acid in the body. This goes for decaf too, if you're concerned about the unwanted effects of caffeine consumption. One study showed that four cups a day lowered the risk of gout in men.

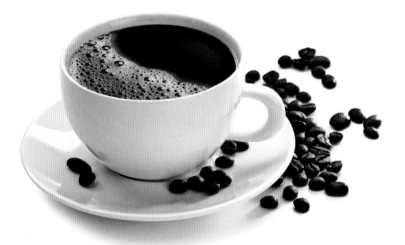

❧ HANGNAILS ❧

Those tiny pieces of torn skin hanging from your cuticles can be a real pain. Hangnails are frequently caused by picking the skin around or biting your nails, or sometimes by dryness or chemicals in soaps and dish detergents. In addition to being unattractive, hangnails can hurt, bleed, and even get infected. To prevent hangnails, keeping your hands moisturized is a good start. But should you find yourself with painful hangnails, don't worry—simple, natural treatments are at your fingertips.

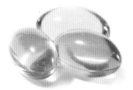

Vitamin E Oil

Vitamin E oil is quickly absorbed by the skin and promotes healing. Apply the oil several times a day; once the hangnail is softened, you can trim it with a cuticle scissor.

Honey

Honey is an intense natural moisturizer with anti-inflammatory and antibacterial properties. Rub a little honey on your hangnails and leave on for a few hours, or, to prevent hangnails, apply periodically to cuticles.

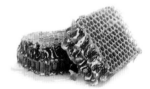

HANGNAILS AND INFECTION

On occasion, bacteria from the air or the mouth (when someone tries to bite off the hangnail) can cause an infection. If an infection occurs, you may notice swelling, redness, and discharge from the area. Soak your finger in warm, salty water and apply antibacterial ointments. If the symptoms continue, seek medical attention, as you may need antibiotics.

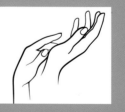

Petroleum Jelly

Packed with good fats offering powerful skin hydration, petroleum jelly is a messy but effective treatment for hangnails. Spread petroleum jelly on your nails before going to bed, and rinse off in the morning.

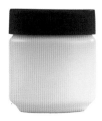

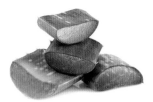

Aloe Vera

Aloe vera gel moisturizes and heals skin, has antimicrobial properties to help prevent infection, and can help dull the pain of a hangnail. Apply the gel from an aloe vera plant to the affected area; leave on for fifteen minutes and then rinse off the excess gel. Repeat daily as needed.

Avocado

Rich in vitamin E, avocados can moisturize and repair those hangnails. Add 2 tablespoons of coconut oil—another great moisturizer with antibacterial and antifungal properties to prevent infection—to mashed-up avocado flesh and apply the moisturizer to your nails at bedtime. Rinse off in the morning; repeat several times a week.

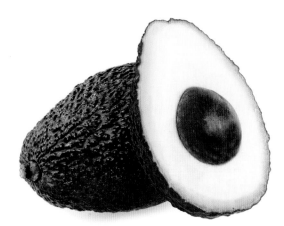

❧ HANGOVER ❧

You may not remember much about last night, but this morning is proving to be pretty unforgettable—and for all the wrong reasons. When you overindulge in alcohol, you may find yourself paying for it later, with symptoms including nausea, vomiting, headaches, dizziness, and more. Alcohol can play havoc with your body, causing dehydration, irritating your stomach lining, and lowering your blood sugar level, leading to exhaustion and fatigue. The way to avoid a hangover is quite simple—don't drink. If you do drink, do so in moderation and on a full stomach. While hangovers usually go away on their own within twenty-four hours, getting through that time period can be challenging. Try the following remedies to ease the pain of a night out gone wrong.

WHEN ALCOHOL IS POISON

Alcohol poisoning is a dangerous, life-threatening condition that needs immediate medical treatment. Symptoms may include:

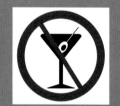

- Irregular breathing

- Mental confusion, stupor, or coma

- Vomiting

- Cold, clammy skin

- Seizures

- Passing out

- Inability to rouse from unconsciousness

If someone is showing any of these signs—or if the person is responding to alcohol in any way that you find unusual or worrisome, call 911. You could save a life.

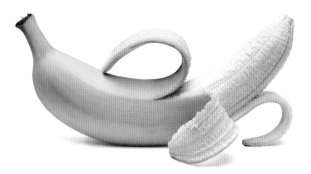

Bananas

Alcohol consumption is typically accompanied by frequent urination, leading to a loss of valuable potassium and causing weakness and fatigue. Give yourself an energy boost with a potassium-loaded banana when you wake up—or, to help prevent some hangover symptoms, have a banana before going to bed after drinking.

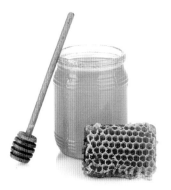

Honey

The fructose in honey can help your body metabolize all that alcohol. According to scientists at the Royal Society of Chemistry in the UK, your body converts alcohol into acetaldehyde, a toxic chemical contributing to your morning-after nausea and headaches. Fructose helps convert acetaldehyde into less-painful chemicals burned during normal metabolic processes. You can eat plain honey, or serve some up on toast to replenish lost sodium and potassium as well.

Fruit Juice

Similar to honey, fruit juices such as apple or cranberry juice contain fructose to help metabolize alcohol. They also can replenish lost vitamins and rehydrate your body.

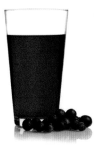

❧ HEADACHES ❧

Whether it's a sharp twinge, an incessant throb, or a dull ache, a headache is a real pain. *Tension headaches* are the most common, characterized by dull pain and pressure. *Migraine headaches* tend to be throbbing and intense, and are often accompanied by other symptoms such as nausea and sensitivity to light. *Cluster headache*s, with severe, recurring pain typically around the eye, are perhaps the most excruciating form of headache.

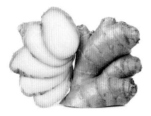

Ginger

Ginger is great at reducing inflammation, and can also help eliminate nausea—making it a good fit for migraine sufferers. To make ginger tea, combine twelve slices of ginger with 3 cups of water in a pot and simmer for twenty minutes. Remove from heat, strain, and drink when warm.

Caffeine

Caffeine can constrict swollen blood vessels in the head, offering some pain relief. In fact, caffeine is found in many over-the-counter headache medicines. Sip caffeinated coffee or soda slowly for headache relief. But, if you're a heavy drinker of caffeinated beverages like coffee or soda, then this remedy isn't for you. Too much caffeine can actually make headaches worse—as can a sudden decrease in caffeine from quitting cold turkey.

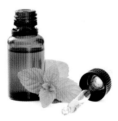

Peppermint Oil

Great for tension headaches, peppermint oil relaxes head and neck muscles. Apply it directly to your hairline for relief (do not apply on an infant or young child).

Heat and Cold

If tightness in your neck is causing your headache, a warm compress can ease the tension and relieve pain. For the throbbing pain of a migraine, try applying a cold compress to your temples. This can cool the artery supplying blood to the lining of the brain and ease the throbbing.

MIGRAINE HEADACHES

According to the World Health Organization, migraines affect at least one adult in every seven in the world. Migraine sufferers typically experience severe pain in one area of the head, along with nausea, blurred vision, and sensitivity to light and sound. Sometimes migraines are preceded by *auras*, or visual 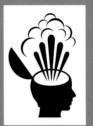 disturbances such as flashes of light or bright spots. An attack can last for hours or days.

Scientists aren't sure what cause migraines, although there are various theories about genetics, blood vessel problems, and underlying central nervous system disorders. There are, however, certain triggers that seem to be common among sufferers:

- Certain foods, including aged cheeses, chocolates, and foods containing nitrites and nitrates (such as hot dogs)

- Food additives such as aspartame or MSG

- Excessive amounts of caffeine

- Alcohol

- Menstruation

- Stress

- Changes in the weather

If you suffer from migraines, keep a record of what foods, environmental changes, and other factors precede the attacks. Avoiding triggers is often your best defense against migraines. Should you get a headache, talk to your doctor and try the home remedies listed above.

❧ HEARTBURN ❧

You've just had a big meal and now your chest is aflame. You go to lie down, thinking rest may help—only to find you feel suddenly worse. Chances are something you ate triggered heartburn, a painful condition where acid in the stomach makes its way back up to the esophagus (a process known as *acid reflux*). This reflux is often worse when you bend over or lie down. Over-the-counter medications such as antacids can often neutralize stomach acid. If you prefer a natural approach, consider the remedies and lifestyle changes below.

WARNING

If you experience heartburn more than twice a week, and neither the remedies listed here nor over-the-counter medications relieve your symptoms, consult a doctor. You may have a condition known as gastroesophageal reflux disease, or GERD. Also call your doctor immediately if the chest pain is severe or accompanied by signs of a heart attack, such as shortness of breath, pain in the arm or jaw, heavy sweating, or light-headedness.

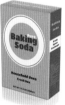

Baking Soda

Sodium bicarbonate, or baking soda, acts as an antacid, neutralizing stomach acid and easing your heartburn. Mix half a teaspoon of baking soda in a glass of water, and drink every two hours. Baking soda is high in salt, however, so if you have frequent heartburn, consult your doctor about alternatives.

Gum

According to a study published in the *Journal of Dental Research*, of thirty-one patients with acid reflux, chewing sugarless gum for half an hour after a meal reduced painful acid reflux. The reasoning is that chewing gum increases saliva production, which neutralizes and washes away acids, and speeds up digestion, giving acids less time to hang out in the esophagus and stomach.

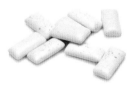

AVOID THE BURN

Certain foods may contribute to heartburn. Avoid these common triggers:

- Fatty foods

- Peppermint

- Chocolate

- Black pepper and other spicy foods

- Citrus fruits

Also avoid alcohol, caffeinated beverages, and eating too close to bedtime.

Apple Cider Vinegar

It's not entirely clear why acidic apple cider vinegar would help relieve acid reflux. But many people swear by this remedy. One theory is that having too little acid in the stomach can trigger the muscle that controls the esophageal opening to loosen, allowing for reflux. Whatever the reason, this is a popular remedy: just pour a teaspoon of apple cider vinegar in a glass half-filled with water and sip.

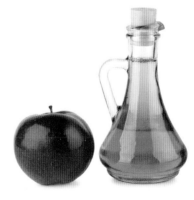

❧ HEMORRHOIDS ❧

While they may be embarrassing to talk about, around 75 percent of people will have hemorrhoids at some point in their lives, according to the National Institute of Diabetes and Digestive and Kidney Diseases. Hemorrhoids occur when veins around the anus or in the lower rectum become swollen and inflamed. While hemorrhoids are generally not dangerous, they can cause discomfort, itching, pain, and bleeding. Hemorrhoids are common during pregnancy, due to hormonal changes, pressure from the growing uterus, and constipation (and consequent straining in the bathroom). Treatments may include over-the-counter creams and suppositories, various outpatient procedures at your doctor's office, or, in severe cases, surgery.

Home treatments for hemorrhoids are relatively simple. Often a change in diet, along with increased water and exercise, can ease the problem. Several natural remedies can relieve the discomfort of hemorrhoids as well.

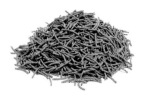

Fiber

Eating foods rich in fiber can soften your stools and reduce strain during bowel movements. A high-fiber diet includes whole grains, beans, fruits such as raspberries and pears, and vegetables such as celery, carrots, and broccoli.

Witch Hazel

Witch hazel can shrink and contract blood vessels, easing the swelling and pain of hemorrhoids. Use a cotton ball to apply the witch hazel directly to the rectum.

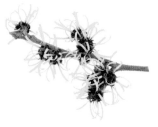

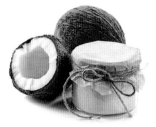

Coconut Oil

With its anti-inflammatory and soothing properties, coconut oil can help to shrink and relieve the discomfort of hemorrhoids. Apply the coconut oil directly to the hemorrhoid. Repeat this process several times a day.

DIABETICS BEWARE

For those suffering from diabetes—including pregnant women with gestational diabetes—certain over-the-counter creams and suppositories may be a risk. That's because they may contain steroids or other ingredients that can cause blood sugar to rise. If you're diabetic and dealing with hemorrhoids, consider natural alternatives to these medications, and be sure to discuss any potential treatment with your doctor.

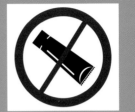

Sitz Baths

To increase blood flow and relieve the irritation of hemorrhoids, try a sitz bath. Fill a bathtub with 3–4 inches of warm water, and soak for fifteen to twenty minutes several times a day, including after each bowel movement. Gently pat dry with a towel when you are done. You can also purchase a special tub that fits over a toilet seat if that's more comfortable for you.

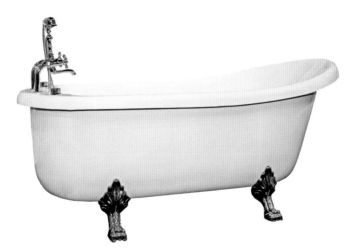

❧ HICCUPS ❧

Hiccups are involuntary contractions of the diaphragm, followed by a quick closing of the vocal cords. Suddenly, your conversation is punctuated with uncontrollable and embarrassing "hic" noises that seem to go on forever (although generally only last a few minutes). While scientists are unsure what causes hiccups, there do seem to be some consistent triggers, such as alcohol or carbonated drinks, spicy food, large meals, or even excitement. While hiccups usually subside on their own without treatment, try the following tips and tricks to end a bout of hiccups—*fast!*

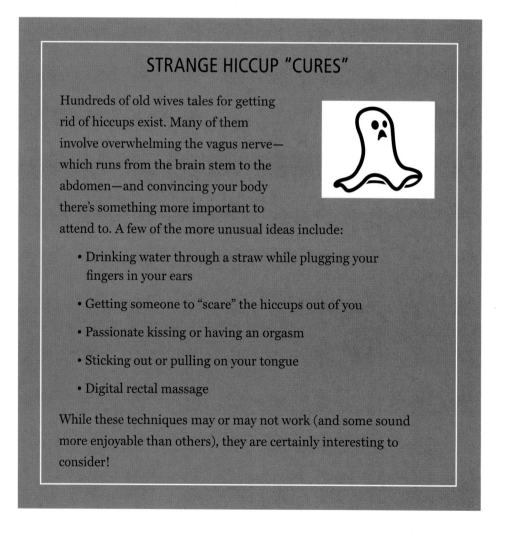

STRANGE HICCUP "CURES"

Hundreds of old wives tales for getting rid of hiccups exist. Many of them involve overwhelming the vagus nerve—which runs from the brain stem to the abdomen—and convincing your body there's something more important to attend to. A few of the more unusual ideas include:

- Drinking water through a straw while plugging your fingers in your ears

- Getting someone to "scare" the hiccups out of you

- Passionate kissing or having an orgasm

- Sticking out or pulling on your tongue

- Digital rectal massage

While these techniques may or may not work (and some sound more enjoyable than others), they are certainly interesting to consider!

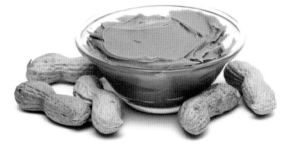

Peanut Butter

Try eating a teaspoon of peanut butter. The lengthy, involved process of chewing and swallowing something sticky like peanut butter may disrupt a hiccup cycle.

Sugar

A spoonful of sugar may make the medicine go down, but a teaspoon full of sugar may end an annoying bout of hiccups. Sugar may stimulate the vagus nerve, which carries signals to the brain, and "distract" your body from hiccupping. Swallow it straight, without mixing it with water or other ingredients.

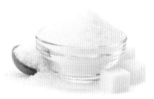

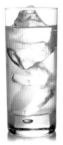

Water

Swallowing water may interrupt the spasmodic cycle of hiccups. You can also try drinking the water upside-down to stimulate the nerves in the back of the throat, and potentially disrupt nerve impulses making you hiccup.

Hold Your Breath

Another theory suggests that increasing your carbon dioxide levels can eliminate hiccups by getting your body to focus on exhaling the carbon dioxide. There are various techniques you can try, such as holding your breath as long as possible, breathing into a paper bag, or inhaling a series of breaths before exhaling.

❧ HIGH BLOOD PRESSURE ❧

Also known as hypertension, high blood pressure occurs when blood flows through your arteries with enough force to cause damage. This high pressure leads to a thickening of the artery walls, and can increase your risk of clots, stroke, and heart and kidney disease. Normal blood pressure is 120/80 millimeters of mercury (mm Hg) or below. When the systolic (top) number rises to 140, or the diastolic (bottom) number reaches 90, your doctor will probably diagnose you with high blood pressure. While it's often difficult to pinpoint hypertension's exact cause, contributing factors may include a high-salt diet, smoking, excessive alcohol consumption, and lack of exercise. While high blood pressure should be monitored by a physician who may prescribe medication, diet and lifestyle choices can go a long way toward managing hypertension.

DASH

Short for Dietary Approaches to Stop Hypertension, this diet is specially designed to lower blood pressure. The DASH diet emphasizes fruits and vegetables, whole grains, low-fat dairy, and lean meats. To determine the right amount of servings for you, visit the National Heart, Lung, and Blood Institute, which offers a special pamphlet on this diet: http://www.nhlbi.nih.gov/files/docs/public/heart/dash_brief.pdf

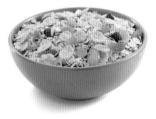

Oat Cereal

In a 2002 study published in the *Journal of Family Practice*, participants who ate fiber-rich whole oat cereal experienced a 7.5 mm Hg drop in systolic blood pressure and a 5.5 mm Hg reduction in diastolic pressure. To reap the benefits of the soluble fiber in oats, known as beta-glucan, add a bowl of oat cereal to your breakfast each morning.

BY THE NUMBERS

According to the American Heart Association, there is an alarming increase in high blood pressure—and related fatalities—in the U.S. Between 2001 and 2011, the annual number of deaths related to high blood pressure rose 39 percent, and 41 percent of American adults are expected to have high blood pressure by 2030.

Garlic

According to various studies, garlic can lower blood pressure due to an active ingredient called allicin, which stimulates production of nitric oxide and hydrogen sulfide, helping to relax blood vessels. However, according to a review of twenty-one studies, supplements work better than raw garlic (and smell better too). Look for a supplement with an allicin yield of 1.8 milligrams per dose.

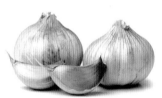

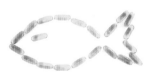

Fish Oil

The omega-3 fatty acids found in certain fish, such as sardines, tuna, and mackerel, can help to lower blood pressure. Add two servings of fish a week to your diet or fish oil capsules to your supplement regimen. Recommended supplement dosages vary widely, so consult a doctor on the appropriate of amount of DHA and EPA for you.

❧ HIGH CHOLESTEROL ❧

Cholesterol gets a bad rap. Your body needs a certain amount of cholesterol—a waxy substance found in cells—to perform important functions from maintaining cell membranes to synthesizing sex hormones. Things go wrong, however, when you have too much cholesterol, especially the "bad" type, or low-density lipoprotein (LDL) cholesterol. When LDL cholesterol levels are too high, fatty deposits called plaque may form on the walls of your arteries, restricting the flow of oxygen and placing you at risk of heart attack or stroke. High cholesterol generally has no symptoms and is detected by your doctor through a blood test. While genetics can play a role in high cholesterol, many lifestyle choices factor in as well, such as poor diet, lack of exercise, and obesity. Your doctor may prescribe medications to lower your cholesterol, however you also should consider diet and lifestyle changes.

Fish

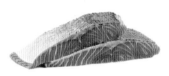

Omega-3 fatty acids can lower your levels of LDL cholesterol and harmful triglycerides. Add two servings of salmon, sardines, tuna, mackerel, or other fish to your diet each week. If you opt for a fish oil supplement, recommended dosages vary, so consult a doctor on the appropriate of amount of DHA and EPA for you.

FISH AND MERCURY

According to the US Environmental Protection Agency (EPA), nearly all fish and shellfish contain traces of mercury. While the amounts are generally not harmful to most people, pregnant women, nursing mothers, and young children need to take special care and avoid fish known to be high in mercury, such as shark, swordfish, king mackerel, and tilefish. Lower-mercury options include shrimp or salmon. Always talk to your doctor about your diet if you're pregnant or nursing.

Olive Oil

Rich in antioxidants, olive oil lowers LDL cholesterol, while not affecting the "good" high-density lipoprotein (HDL) cholesterol that removes LDL cholesterol from your arteries. Try replacing butter and other dietary fats with 2 tablespoons of extra virgin olive oil a day.

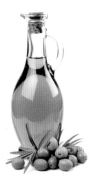

Fiber

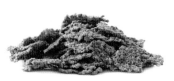

There are different theories as to how fiber lowers LDL cholesterol levels. Some believe it binds to cholesterol in the digestive system, preventing it from being absorbed in the body. Others speculate it takes the place of higher-cholesterol foods in the diet. No matter the reason, fiber has been shown to reduce bad cholesterol levels. So add some high-fiber foods to your diet, including whole grains, beans, fruits, and vegetables. Black beans are especially high in fiber.

Nuts

Nuts are rich in saturated and polyunsaturated "good" fats that, when consumed in place of saturated fats (such as cheese or cream) can help lower LDL cholesterol levels and keep arteries healthy.

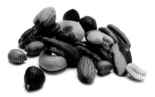

Avocado

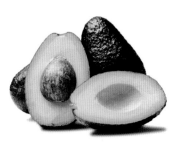

Rich in vitamins, minerals, and monounsaturated fats that help lower bad cholesterol in the blood, avocados are a tasty way to lower your cholesterol. According to a recent study in the *Journal of the American Heart Association,* eating one avocado a day significantly reduced participants' LDL cholesterol levels. Since avocados are caloric, limit yourself to one a day.

❧ HIVES ❧

People who get hives know the itch well. Also called urticaria, hives are raised pink or red welts that can be small spots or several inches across, sometimes connecting together to form larger welts. While a single hive may go away in twenty-four hours, others may then appear, meaning an outbreak of hives can last for days or even longer. According to the American Academy of Dermatology, hives can be triggered by allergic reactions to foods, such as citrus fruits, milk, nuts, or fish, medications, pollen, insect bites, or other allergens. They can also be triggered by stress, sunlight, or certain illnesses. While hives typically resolve without treatment, your doctor may recommend an over-the-counter antihistamine to relieve the itch. Or, you can try one of the below home remedies to give your skin a break.

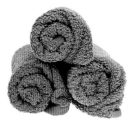

Cold Compress

Since heat and excitement can trigger or worsen hives, use a cold compress to soothe your skin and relieve the itch. The cold will shrink blood vessels and numb the skin slightly. Apply for ten minutes at a time.

Oatmeal

To relieve itch, bathe in colloidal (or finely ground) oatmeal, available at your local drugstore. Or, make your own colloidal oatmeal by placing 2 cups of oatmeal in a blender, and blending until it forms a fine powder. Sprinkle the oatmeal in lukewarm bathwater and soak for ten to fifteen minutes.

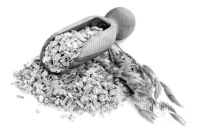

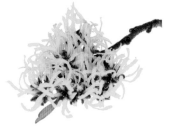

Witch Hazel

With anti-inflammatory and astringent properties, witch hazel is used for various skin conditions. Apply witch hazel directly to the welts for relief.

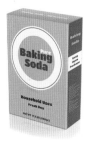

Baking Soda

Baking soda can relieve itching. Sprinkle it in your bath, or mix 1 teaspoon of baking soda in 4 ounces of water and apply the mixture directly to the affected area.

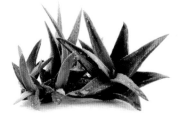

Aloe Vera

The soothing, anti-inflammatory properties of aloe vera can relieve the itch of hives. Apply the gel from an aloe vera plant directly to your hives. (You can use an aloe vera cream if necessary, but the gel from a plant will work better.)

Milk of Magnesia

The alkaline nature of milk of magnesia will stop itch in its tracks. Dab some on your hives for quick relief.

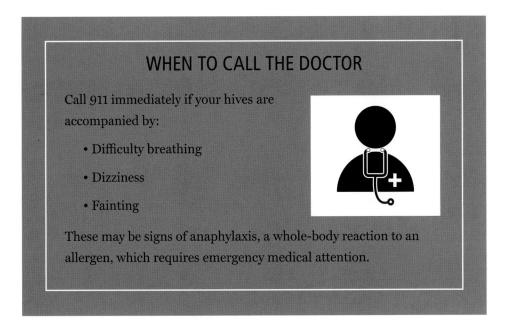

WHEN TO CALL THE DOCTOR

Call 911 immediately if your hives are accompanied by:

- Difficulty breathing

- Dizziness

- Fainting

These may be signs of anaphylaxis, a whole-body reaction to an allergen, which requires emergency medical attention.

❧ HOT FLASHES ❧

When women approach menopause with a sense of foreboding, it's usually because of hot flashes. This common symptom of menopause involves sudden warmth on the face, neck, and chest. While hot flashes generally aren't serious, they can be extremely uncomfortable and tend to be worse at night, causing sweats, chills, and sleeplessness. While doctors sometimes use hormone therapy (estrogen and progesterone) to treat hot flashes, this may cause other health complications. As an alternative, consider these natural treatments to turn down the heat—and finally get a good night's sleep.

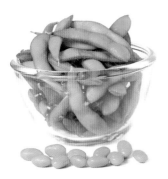

Soy

Soy contains estrogen-like compounds and is a staple in Asian countries, where menopausal women report fewer hot flashes than in the United States. While studies have been mixed over the years as to how well soy works to eliminate hot flashes, researchers recently reviewed nineteen studies comparing soy to a placebo, and found that it may indeed help relieve hot flashes over time. Add two servings of soy to your diet a day; popular options include edamame, soy milk, and tofu.

HOT HABITS TO BREAK

To turn down the thermostat, avoid these hot-flash triggers:

- Alcohol

- Caffeinated beverages

- Smoking

- Hot, spicy foods

Losing weight and exercising also can reduce your hot flashes—and keep the rest of you healthy as well.

Black Cohosh

Also known as black snakeroot or bugbane, black cohosh is a root that affects the endocrine system. While it's unclear exactly how it works, it's a popular treatment for symptoms of menopause, and is approved by the German government as an alternative to hormone therapy. Extracts are available at health food stores, often as 20-milligram pills taken twice a day (although follow the label instructions regarding dosage).

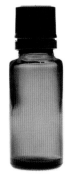

WARNING

Talk to your doctor if you're considering taking black cohosh, as there have been questions about the root's effect on the liver.

Flaxseed

With natural plant estrogens, flaxseed is another alternative to taking estrogen. A small pilot study conducted by Mayo Clinic researchers found that women who ate flaxseed experienced a 50 percent decrease in hot flashes. While further studies are necessary to confirm flaxseed's effectiveness in treating hot flashes, it's certainly worth a try. Study participants consumed 4 tablespoons of ground flaxseed a day; however, to prevent indigestion, try starting with 2 tablespoons and working your way up. You can add ground flaxseed to yogurt, hot cereal, or smoothies.

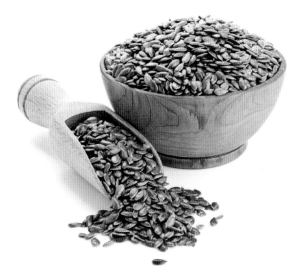

✍ IMPOTENCE ✍

While it may "happen to every man," when it starts happening more often, erectile dysfunction, or impotence, can be a real problem. Impotence refers to difficulty getting or maintaining an erection, and can be caused by physical and/or psychological factors. Sometimes, impotence is the result of a medical condition such as heart disease, diabetes, or high blood pressure, or is a side effect of prescription medications. Other times it's caused by anxiety, depression, or issues within a relationship. Certain lifestyle factors, such as obesity, fatigue, smoking, or alcohol use, can also contribute to erectile dysfunction. Various well-advertised prescription treatments exist for impotence; however, if you prefer to go the natural route, try these home remedies to address this frustrating problem.

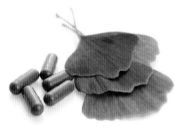

Ginkgo

Ginkgo biloba, used in Chinese medicine, is popular alternative treatment for impotence, due to its supposed ability to improve blood flow. Ginkgo is available as a supplement, with recommended dosages up to 240 milligrams a day. Ginkgo may interfere with certain medications, so talk to your doctor before beginning a supplement.

Ginseng

A 2008 review of various clinical studies showed that Korean red ginseng—also known as Asian ginseng—may help treat erectile dysfunction. The root of the Korean ginseng plant is believed to improve energy and blood flow to the penis. Red ginseng supplements are available at health food stores; follow the label for the correct dosage. Talk to your doctor before beginning a supplement, as red ginseng may interfere with certain medications, including blood thinners and insulin.

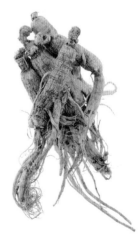

LESS WEIGHT, MORE SATISFACTION

If you're overweight and struggling with erectile dysfunction, try shedding some pounds. An Australian study published in the *Journal of Sexual Medicine* found that when obese men with diabetes lost just 5 to 10 percent of their body weight over a two-month period, their erectile function and sexual desire improved. Obesity can affect blood vessels and lower testosterone levels—both of which contribute to impotence. Losing weight can rectify these problems—and give you added energy and self-confidence, which are a big help in the bedroom!

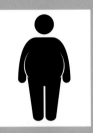

Zinc

Proponents of zinc as a treatment for impotence cite its ability to improve the body's natural testosterone levels, as demonstrated in a 1996 study published in the journal *Nutrition*. Of course, zinc will only help if the cause of your erectile dysfunction is low testosterone—if it's related to disease or lifestyle factors, you'll need to seek an alternative. Dietary zinc is found in beef, pork, chicken, nuts, and whole grains. You can also take a zinc supplement, but do not exceed 40 milligrams a day.

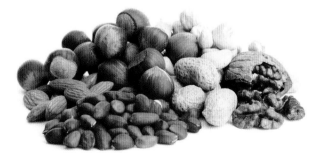

❧ INCONTINENCE ❧

If you suffer from urinary incontinence, you may feel like the only adult in the world incapable of controlling his or her bladder. However, according to the World Health Organization, more than 200 million people worldwide suffer from this problem, with women suffering at a disproportionate rate. There are different types of incontinence: With *stress incontinence*, actions such as laughing, coughing, or sneezing cause you to leak fluid. With *urge incontinence*, also known as overactive bladder, you feel a sudden and uncontrollable need to urinate. Many factors contribute to incontinence, including pregnancy, childbirth, aging, and various diseases or medical treatments—as well as simple, easily treated conditions such as urinary tract infections. While prescription medications and therapies—as well as surgeries—exist to treat incontinence, you may also consider these natural approaches to keep you dry and accident-free.

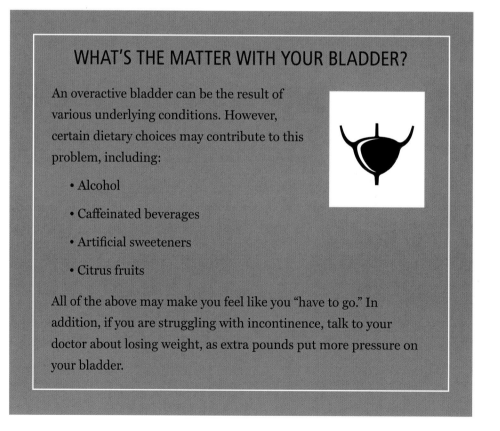

WHAT'S THE MATTER WITH YOUR BLADDER?

An overactive bladder can be the result of various underlying conditions. However, certain dietary choices may contribute to this problem, including:

- Alcohol

- Caffeinated beverages

- Artificial sweeteners

- Citrus fruits

All of the above may make you feel like you "have to go." In addition, if you are struggling with incontinence, talk to your doctor about losing weight, as extra pounds put more pressure on your bladder.

Vitamin D

Vitamin D deficiency may be tied to pelvic floor disorders such as urinary incontinence, according to a 2010 study reported in *Obstetrics and Gynecology*. You can find vitamin D, essential for bone and muscle strength, in fortified milk, eggs, and fatty fish.

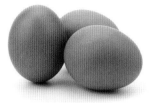

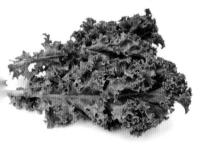

Magnesium

In a double-blind study, women who took 150 milligrams of magnesium twice a day experienced fewer episodes of urge incontinence and waking at night to urinate. One thought is that magnesium relieves muscle spasms of the bladder. Magnesium is found in dark leafy greens, nuts, and beans, or you can take supplements (150 milligrams, twice a day).

Exercises

Pregnant women or women who've recently given birth are often advised by doctors to do Kegel exercises, a type of activity designed to strengthen your pelvic floor muscles. These exercises basically involve squeezing the muscles you use to hold your urine. Start by squeezing for three seconds, and then releasing for three seconds. Do ten repetitions, three times a day. Each week, add seconds until you're squeezing for ten seconds at a time.

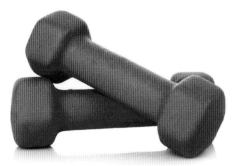

❧ INGROWN HAIRS ❧

Is that strange bump on your face a pimple? Or is it an ingrown hair? Ingrown hairs occur when hair curls back into the skin instead of growing out of it. Ingrown hairs may look a little like pimples or be filled with pus, and can result in irritation, pain, and inflammation. They are often caused by closely shaving or tweezing hair, or sometimes by dead skin obscuring hair follicles. They mostly affect men with coarse or curly hair, appearing on the beard area, although women may get ingrown hairs in areas they frequently shave as well, such as the armpits, legs, and pubic area. Ingrown hairs are rarely serious. If not shaving isn't feasible, then consider these home remedies to smooth out this hairy situation.

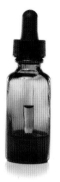

Tea Tree Oil

Tea tree oil has anti-inflammatory and antibacterial properties that can help heal an ingrown hair and keep infection at bay. Dilute the oil, using a ratio of one part oil to nine parts water. If you find this makes your skin too dry, mix a couple drops of tea tree oil in 2–3 teaspoons of skin-soothing aloe vera instead. Use a cotton ball to apply the oil to the affected area, twice a day until symptoms subside.

Sugar

Sugar naturally exfoliates the skin, removing dead cells so that the ingrown hair can reach the surface. Mix equal parts sugar and olive oil or honey to form a paste. (Olive oil is a powerful moisturizer, and honey has antibacterial and pain-relieving properties.) Apply this paste to the affected area, and scrub gently in a circular motion to loosen the dead skin; after a few minutes, wipe the paste off with warm water.

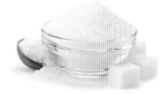

WATCH HOW YOU SHAVE

To avoid ingrown hairs, try adjusting how you shave. Avoid shaving too close and putting too much pressure on the blade. Shave in the direction of the hair, and use a single-blade razor. And, to soften the hair before shaving, first prep the area by applying a warm washcloth for several minutes.

Tweezers

The most common treatment is physical removal of the ingrown hair, provided it's near the surface where you can see it. Soften the skin for several minutes with a warm washcloth then use a sterilized needle or tweezers to pluck the ingrown hair. Immediately disinfect the area afterward with rubbing alcohol or another antiseptic.

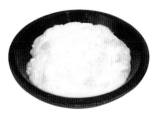

Baking Soda

Baking soda has anti-inflammatory properties and can exfoliate the skin, relieving the pain, redness, and swelling of an ingrown hair. Mix 1 tablespoon of baking soda with 1 cup of water, and apply the mixture to your skin with a cotton ball. Rinse off after five minutes with cold water.

❧ INSECT BITES AND STINGS ❧

Insect bites and stings are the bane of summertime. They can distract from a family picnic, or ruin an afternoon hike. When a mosquito, spider, tick, bee, or other insect gets you, they inject poison or another harmful substance into your skin. You may feel the pain immediately, such as with a bee sting, or you may not realize you've been bitten until later, such as when you experience the swelling and itch of a mosquito bite. Generally, insect bites resolve on their own within a few days. However, some people experience allergic reactions to bites and stings, which can be intense or even life-threatening. For more mild cases, try these natural approaches to take the pain out of a bite or a sting.

WARNING

Some people develop anaphylaxis, a whole-body reaction to an allergen, from insect bites and stings. Call 911 if a bite or sting is accompanied by difficulty breathing, dizziness, fainting, facial swelling, or vomiting.

Ice

Ice numbs pain and decreases the release of itch-causing histamines. Apply on and off for ten minutes at a time until you feel relief. Make sure to wrap the ice in a cloth; do not apply directly to the skin.

Tea Tree Oil

Antibacterial tea tree oil can relieve itching. Dilute the oil, using a ratio of one part oil to nine parts water. Use a cotton ball to apply the oil to the affected area, twice a day until you feel better. If tea tree oil is too harsh for your skin, even diluted, you can try coconut oil instead, which also has antibacterial and soothing properties.

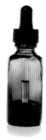

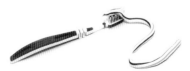

Toothpaste

Mint or peppermint-flavored toothpaste can cool an itchy bite. Apply a small amount directly to the bite for relief.

Baking Soda

Baking soda eases inflammation and itchiness. Add water to baking soda until it forms a paste and apply to the site of the bite or sting for twenty to thirty minutes.

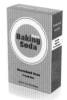

WHAT BIT YOU?

When it comes to treating bites and stings, it's important to know what got you.

Bees: If you've been stung by a bee, remove the stinger as quickly as possible. You can do this with your fingernails or a pair of tweezers, or use the edge of a credit card to scrape out the stinger. Wash the area with soap and water, and use one of the methods listed here for pain relief.

Spiders: Most spiders are not dangerous. Unless you've been bitten by a poisonous spider such as the black widow or brown recluse spider in the U.S., clean the wound with soap and water and apply an antiseptic ointment. Treat any discomfort with the methods listed here. If the bite is accompanied by severe pain, difficulty breathing, or other worrisome symptoms, seek immediate medical attention.

Ticks: While tick bites aren't generally harmful, Lyme disease is always a concern. If you've been bitten, use tweezers to ease the tick out carefully without crushing it or leaving any part of it in your skin. Keep the tick in a sealed container if possible to show a doctor should you develop symptoms of Lyme disease, such as a rash with a bull's-eye pattern, fever, chills, or muscle pain.

Regardless of the type of bite or sting, if you have allergies or experience signs of anaphylaxis (see the warning on the previous page), seek immediate medical attention.

❦ INSOMNIA ❦

Does this scenario sound familiar? You lay awake, mind racing, unable to fall asleep. As the minutes, or hours, tick by you become increasingly anxious about sleeping— making it even harder to drift off to sleep. If you have difficulty falling or staying asleep three or more nights a week, you may have insomnia. Insomnia can lead to irritability, anxiety, or depression, as well as poor performance at work, difficulty making decisions, and a general lack of focus. Causes are diverse, and may include stress, anxiety, or depression; too much caffeine during the day; irregular sleep habits; certain medications; and age-related conditions such as arthritis, in which pain or discomfort may interfere with sleep. While doctors sometimes prescribe medications to help you sleep, you can also try natural approaches to help you get your zzzs.

TURN OFF THAT TABLET

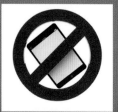

Studies have shown that the blue lights of many tablets, laptops, smartphones, and certain televisions can make us more alert and interfere with the production of melatonin, a hormone that regulates sleep. As the American Medical Association warns, "exposure to excessive light at night, including extended use of various electronic media, can disrupt sleep or exacerbate sleep disorders, especially in children and adolescents." So if you're having trouble sleeping, make sure to turn off your devices at least two hours before bedtime. Instead, try meditation, yoga, or a warm bath to help you settle down and relax.

Valerian

Medicinal use of this herb dates back to the time of Hippocrates, and it was prescribed for insomnia as early as the second century. Today valerian is available as a dietary supplement and is a common ingredient in many sleep aids. While there is no standard dosage, in studies participants were given 400 to 900 milligrams of valerian extract. Talk to your doctor before taking valerian, as long-term use may be connected to liver damage.

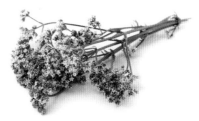

Meditation

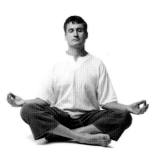

If your sleeplessness is related to anxiety or stress, try adding meditation to your treatment regimen. Meditation can lower blood pressure, improve concentration, and reduce physical and emotional reactions to stress. Sit on a chair with your back straight and your feet flat on the floor, your arms on your thighs with your palms turned upward. (Or, you can assume the traditional lotus position). Breathe regularly by inhaling for six to eight counts, and then holding and exhaling to the same count. Follow these steps daily, gradually increasing the duration of your practice.

Lavender

Lavender is thought to have mild sedative powers. Spray some on your pillow, dab some lavender oil on your temples before bedtime, or add lavender oil to your bath and enjoy a warm, sleep-inducing soak.

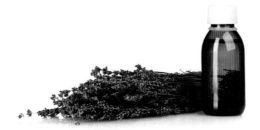

➤ IRRITABLE BOWEL SYNDROME ➤

Irritable bowel syndrome, or IBS, is a chronic condition affecting the large intestine. While people may not like to talk about its unpleasant symptoms—bloating, excess gas, abdominal pain, and constipation and/or diarrhea—IBS is relatively common. In fact, according to the International Foundation for Functional Gastrointestinal Disorders, worldwide prevalence rates for IBS range from 9 to 23 percent of a population. No one knows the exact cause of IBS, although a miscommunication between the GI tract and the brain may lead to muscle spasms in the intestines. Triggers of IBS vary from person to person, and may include stress or certain foods. While severe cases of IBS may require medication, most cases are mild enough to be managed with diet, lifestyle changes, and natural alternatives.

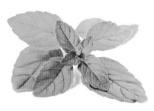

Peppermint

Peppermint can reduce gas and relieve spasms in the gastrointestinal tract. You can buy peppermint tea or make your own by adding dried peppermint leaves to 1 cup of boiled water and steeping for five to ten minutes. Strain and drink 1–2 cups a day. Alternatively, you can take 1–2 enteric-coated capsules, three times a day, about an hour before meals. Talk to your doctor first if you suffer from heartburn.

Fiber

Fiber is tricky for IBS sufferers. While it can ease constipation, too much fiber can worsen gas and abdominal pain. Add fiber to your diet gradually to help with IBS symptoms. Foods rich in fiber include whole grains, beans, fruits, and vegetables. To avoid increased gas, your doctor may advise you to take a fiber supplement instead.

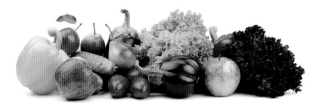

Flaxseed

Ground flaxseed (6–24 grams a day) can help with constipation. According to research reported by the University of Maryland Medical Center, in a study of people with IBS-caused constipation, those who took ground flaxseed reduced constipation, bloating, and abdominal pain more than those who took pysllium, a dietary fiber used as a laxative.

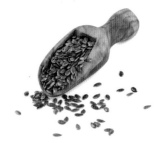

IBS AND DIET

When it comes to IBS and food, everyone differs. You'll need to experiment to see what works for you. Try reducing the following in your diet and see if it makes a difference:

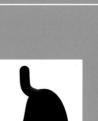

- Caffeine

- Fried foods

- Dairy products

- Chocolate

- Nuts

While increased fiber can help some people, if you find foods such as beans or cauliflower are worsening your gas and bloating, by all means reduce or eliminate them from your diet. Also, try eating smaller, more frequent meals to avoid overwhelming your digestive system.

❧ JET LAG ❧

If you've traveled across multiple time zones, you've probably experienced jet lag. Jet lag occurs when your circadian rhythms—which signal to your body when to sleep and wake—become disturbed. You may experience trouble sleeping, fatigue, problems concentrating, or digestive disturbances. While jet lag is temporary, for each time zone you cross, it can take up to a day to recover. That can really eat into a vacation, or affect your ability to dazzle your audience during a business presentation. While time is the best medicine for jet lag, if you need to quickly adjust to your new schedule, then try these techniques to send your jet lag packing.

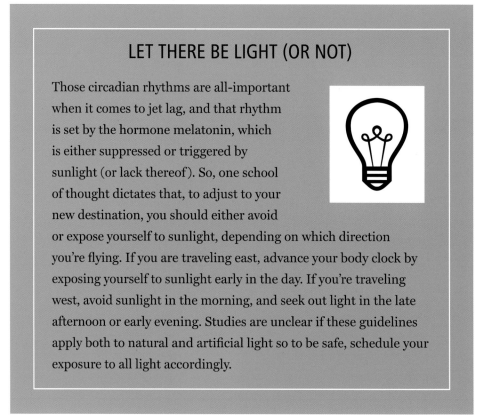

LET THERE BE LIGHT (OR NOT)

Those circadian rhythms are all-important when it comes to jet lag, and that rhythm is set by the hormone melatonin, which is either suppressed or triggered by sunlight (or lack thereof). So, one school of thought dictates that, to adjust to your new destination, you should either avoid or expose yourself to sunlight, depending on which direction you're flying. If you are traveling east, advance your body clock by exposing yourself to sunlight early in the day. If you're traveling west, avoid sunlight in the morning, and seek out light in the late afternoon or early evening. Studies are unclear if these guidelines apply both to natural and artificial light so to be safe, schedule your exposure to all light accordingly.

Melatonin

One of the jobs of this hormone is to manage the body's circadian rhythms. Melatonin cycles are connected to daylight, so if it's light out when you're used to sleeping, you can expect your circadian rhythms to be thrown off. Take 0.5 to 3 milligrams of melatonin an hour or two before bedtime at your destination.

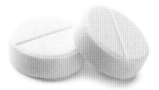

Jump Ahead or Behind

A few days before your trip, start incrementally waking up an hour later or earlier than normal, depending on which direction you're traveling. This gradual adjustment will prepare your body for its new sleep and wake times, so the change won't feel so abrupt when you arrive at your destination.

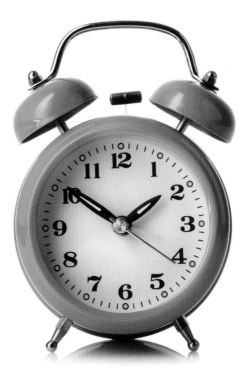

❧ JOCK ITCH ❧

While jock itch may have a humorous name, the itchy, uncomfortable rash is anything but funny to someone experiencing it. Jock itch is generally caused by a fungal infection that spreads from the folds of the groin to the thighs and buttocks, causing pain, itchiness, and sometimes blisters. Jock itch tends to be a complaint of male athletes, and spreads in a similar fashion to athlete's foot, in locker rooms and through use of infected towels or equipment. However, anyone can develop this condition, especially people who are obese or who sweat a lot. Doctors frequently recommend over-the-counter creams for jock itch, sometimes prescribing antifungal creams or pills for more persistent cases that don't respond to home care. For less severe cases, simple home remedies may help ditch the itch.

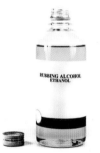

Rubbing Alcohol

Since fungi thrive in wet environments, drying the skin can help to make it less hospitable to these unwelcome visitors. Not only is rubbing alcohol a drying agent, but it can kill fungi on the surface of the skin. Apply to the affected area with a cotton ball after bathing.

Tee Tree Oil

Tea tree oil is antifungal and has anti-inflammatory properties to help soothe your skin. In addition, its antibacterial properties can help prevent a secondary infection. Dilute the oil, using a ratio of one part oil to nine parts water. Use a cotton ball or swab to apply the oil to the affected area twice a day. Or, you can add a few drops of tea tree oil to your bath and soak for ten to fifteen minutes.

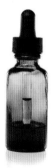

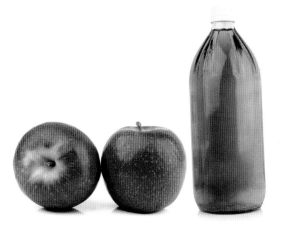

Apple Cider Vinegar

Apple cider vinegar has antifungal, antibacterial, and anti-inflammatory properties, making it a good choice for many skin conditions. Dilute the vinegar, using three parts water to one part ACV, to prevent burning. Wash the rash in this mixture; repeat several times a day.

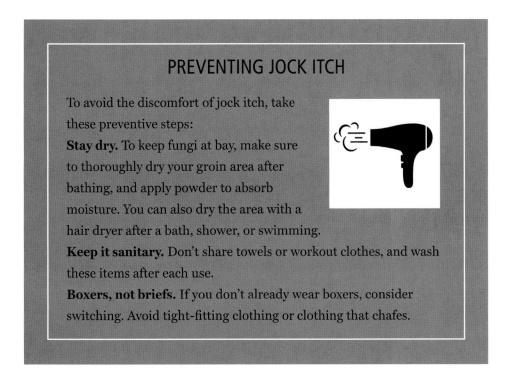

PREVENTING JOCK ITCH

To avoid the discomfort of jock itch, take these preventive steps:

Stay dry. To keep fungi at bay, make sure to thoroughly dry your groin area after bathing, and apply powder to absorb moisture. You can also dry the area with a hair dryer after a bath, shower, or swimming.

Keep it sanitary. Don't share towels or workout clothes, and wash these items after each use.

Boxers, not briefs. If you don't already wear boxers, consider switching. Avoid tight-fitting clothing or clothing that chafes.

❧ KIDNEY STONES ❧

According to the National Kidney Foundation, one in ten people will have a kidney stone in their lifetime. A kidney stone occurs when waste in the urine forms crystals that stay in the kidney or move down the urinary tract. Passing these stones can be painful, and stones that don't move can cause a back-up of urine in the body. If you have kidney stones, you may experience pain on either side of your lower back, blood in your urine, difficulty urinating, cloudy or bad-smelling urine, fever, chills, or vomiting. Causes of kidney stones vary and may include insufficient water intake, urinary tract infections, lack of dietary calcium (or, conversely, too much calcium supplementation), obesity, and eating foods high in purines—such as asparagus, liver, or anchovies—that can lead to a higher production of uric acid. If you have kidney stones, see a doctor as soon as possible; in addition, you can try these home remedies to find some relief.

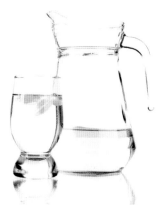

Water

Sometimes drinking plenty of water can flush smaller kidney stones from your body. Drink enough water a day so that your urine is light yellow or clear.

Dandelion Root

Dandelion root may stimulate urine production and cleanse the urinary tract. A typical dosage is 500 milligrams, twice a day.

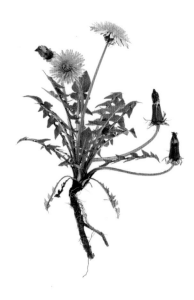

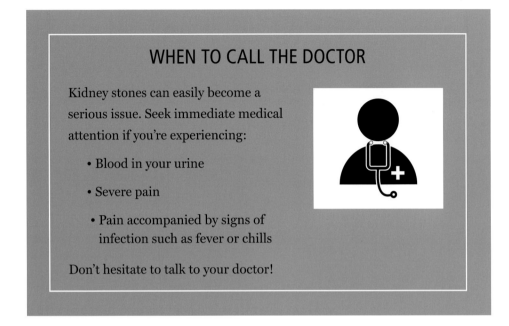

WHEN TO CALL THE DOCTOR

Kidney stones can easily become a serious issue. Seek immediate medical attention if you're experiencing:

- Blood in your urine

- Severe pain

- Pain accompanied by signs of infection such as fever or chills

Don't hesitate to talk to your doctor!

Apple Cider Vinegar

Proponents of this folk remedy claim ACV has an alkalizing effect on the blood and urine, aiding in the digestive process and breaking down kidney stones. Mix 2 teaspoons ACV in 1 cup water, and drink the mixture several times a day.

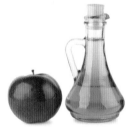

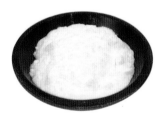

Baking Soda

If you tend to get kidney stones due to uric acid, baking soda may help. Baking soda, or sodium bicarbonate, can help to break up uric acid stones and make the urine less acidic, which may prevent the formation of new stones. Either take sodium bicarbonate tablets (available over the counter), or mix half a teaspoon of baking soda in a glass of water and drink twice a day, between meals.

❧ LARYNGITIS ❧

What was that you said? If you have laryngitis, making yourself heard can be a challenge. Laryngitis is an inflammation of the larynx (or voice box) and vocal chords, making you sound hoarse—if you can be heard at all. It can be caused by overusing your voice (such as shouting at a sporting event), or from a cold, infection, smoking, or gastroesophageal reflux disease (GERD). While "losing your voice" can be frustrating, most cases of laryngitis are temporary and go away on their own within a week or two (if symptoms last longer, consult your doctor). To speed up the healing and regain your voice, try these soothing alternatives.

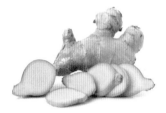

Ginger

With its anti-inflammatory properties, ginger can help relieve the symptoms of laryngitis. Make ginger tea by combining twelve slices of ginger with 3 cups of water in a pot and simmer for twenty minutes. Remove from heat and strain.

KIDS AND CROUP

If your child has symptoms of laryngitis, be sure to keep a careful eye out for signs of croup—a swelling of the voice box and trachea that makes it difficult to breathe. Signs of croup include:

- A bark-like cough

- High-pitch rasping when breathing

- Fever

- Runny nose

- Sore throat

Call the doctor should your child exhibit any of these signs, or if you have any concerns about your child's laryngitis.

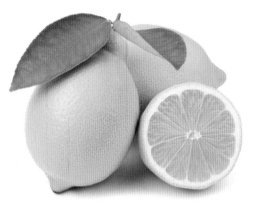

Lemon

The acidity in lemons makes it hard for viruses and bacteria to thrive. Squeeze the juice of a lemon into a bowl, and add a little salt. Add 1 teaspoon of this mixture to 1 cup of warm water and gargle several times a day.

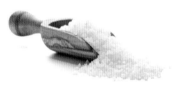

Salt

Salt water can help heal your inflamed vocal cords and relieve the sore throat that often accompanies laryngitis. Dissolve ¼–½ teaspoon of salt in an 8-ounce glass of warm water and briefly gargle several times a day.

Garlic

With its antimicrobial properties, garlic can help with laryngitis caused by bacteria or a virus. Suck on a clove a few times a day, if you can handle the strong taste (and smell!).

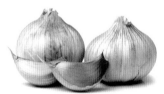

❧ LICE ❧

All parents dread that call from the school nurse, or that letter home notifying them that their child may have been exposed to lice. Lice are tiny insects that live in a person's hair and feed off of small amounts of blood drawn from the scalp. While head lice are common among young children, adults can have lice as well—especially if they have kids. While lice aren't dangerous, they are highly contagious and can cause intense itching. Scratching the scalp can lead to irritation, broken skin, and possible infection. While a number of over-the-counter and prescription lice treatments exist, you may also want to try one of these home remedies to relieve your child of the discomfort of itchy head lice.

Olive Oil

A theory of eliminating lice is that you need to suffocate them. Pour a coat of olive oil over the hair, and use a lice comb (available at drug stores) to comb through a section of hair at a time, removing any lice or their eggs (nits). Rinse with your regular shampoo and repeat the process, doing this every day for a week. Continue using a lice comb daily for the next two to three weeks, making sure the hair is wet and lubricated with conditioner when combing.

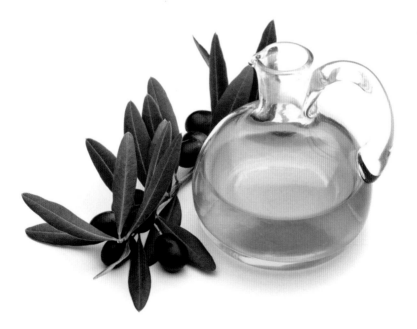

HOW DO LICE SPREAD?

Fortunately, lice can't fly or jump. Instead, they spread through direct contact, or by sharing infected items such as hairbrushes, hats, hair ties, towels, and the like. Encourage your kids not share brushes or other personal items with other children, and reinforce that idea when lice outbreaks occur.

Tea Tree Oil

With its antimicrobial properties, tea tree oil is used to fight various infections and is a common alternative to chemical lice treatments—although experts debate its effectiveness. Add 10 drops of tea tree oil to around ¼ cup of a carrier oil such as olive oil. Coat the hair with this mixture and leave on for two to three hours. Then use a lice comb, soaked in white vinegar (which helps loosen nits from hair shafts), to comb through the hair in sections. Finally rinse out the oil with your regular shampoo. Repeat this process for several days; once you no longer see any nits, continue using the lice comb every three to four days for at least two weeks.

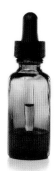

❧ MENSTRUAL CRAMPS ❧

As women around the world know, painful periods can make it difficult to work, focus on school, or get things done around the house. Menstrual cramps, or dysmenorrhea, refer to pain in the abdomen (and often lower back) that women experience around menstruation. Menstrual cramps tend to target women in their teens or twenties, although all pre-menopausal women can be affected. Often menstrual cramps are triggered by hormones, and may lessen with age or after childbirth. In some instances, cramps are caused by underlying conditions, such as fibroids, endometriosis, or pelvic inflammatory disease (PID). While severe cases are sometimes treated with prescription medicines, including birth control pills, menstrual cramps often respond to over-the-counter pain medication such as ibuprofen. If you want to avoid medication, you can also try simple home remedies to ease your monthly pain.

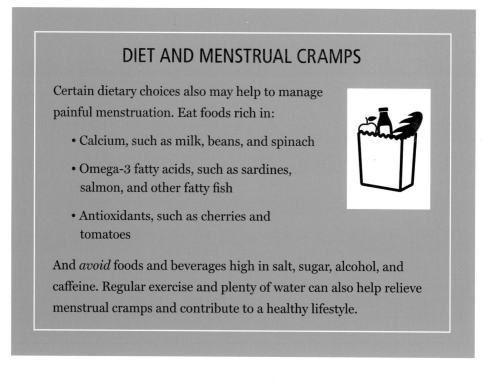

DIET AND MENSTRUAL CRAMPS

Certain dietary choices also may help to manage painful menstruation. Eat foods rich in:

- Calcium, such as milk, beans, and spinach

- Omega-3 fatty acids, such as sardines, salmon, and other fatty fish

- Antioxidants, such as cherries and tomatoes

And *avoid* foods and beverages high in salt, sugar, alcohol, and caffeine. Regular exercise and plenty of water can also help relieve menstrual cramps and contribute to a healthy lifestyle.

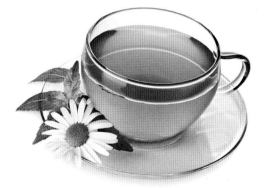

Chamomile Tea

According to a study reported in the American Chemical Society's *Journal of Agricultural and Food Chemistry*, drinking chamomile tea can relieve menstrual cramps. Participants who drank the tea had high levels of glycine in their urine, which is known to relieve muscle spasms and act as a nerve relaxant. Participants drank five cups a day over two weeks.

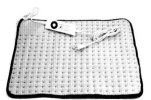

Heat

Painful menstrual cramps can often be relieved with the simple application of heat, which relaxes contracting uterine muscles. Either take a warm bath or use a heating pad, as often as necessary to relieve the pain.

Vitamin D

You may be able to prevent or lessen menstrual cramps by upping your vitamin D intake. According to a study at the University of Messina in Italy, women who took high doses of vitamin D five days before their expected periods reported significantly less pain during menstruation, compared to those who received a placebo. The thinking is that vitamin D inhibits the synthesis of prostaglandin, a hormone responsible for menstrual pain, and also acts as an anti-inflammatory. While exact dosages are still being explored, according to the National Institutes of Health, the recommended daily allowance of vitamin D is 600 IU.

❧ MORNING SICKNESS ❧

There are many joys of pregnancy. Morning sickness, however, is not one of them. It can be hard to get excited about your pregnancy journey when you're feeling nauseous or vomiting day and night. (Unfortunately, despite its moniker, *morning* sickness can occur any time of day.) Fortunately, for many women, morning sickness subsides after the first trimester, although some women may experience this condition throughout their pregnancies. While morning sickness is miserable, it's not generally dangerous. A few basic home remedies can get you back on your feet—and away from the toilet bowl.

Vitamin B6

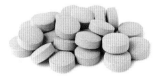

In studies, vitamin B6 has been shown to relieve the symptoms of morning sickness, possibly by helping the body process certain amino acids. The recommended dosage is 100 milligrams or less daily, but, as with all vitamins during pregnancy, consult your doctor to see if vitamin B6 is right for you.

WARNING

If you're pregnant, you should always consult your doctor before taking any herbal supplements, vitamins, or medicines—alternative or otherwise. Your doctor can tell you what's safe for you and your baby.

Ginger

Ginger contains chemicals that ease nausea and inflammation. To make ginger tea, combine twelve slices of ginger with 3 cups of water in a pot and simmer for twenty minutes. Remove from heat and strain. If you're considering taking an herbal ginger supplement, talk to your doctor first. While a recent study showed ginger to be effective in decreasing nausea and vomiting in pregnancy, there are concerns about how it might affect fetal sex hormones.

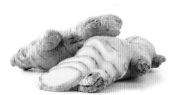

HYPEREMESIS GRAVIDARUM

A small percentage of women experience a more severe form of morning sickness called hyperemesis gravidarum, which sometimes requires hospitalization. According to the American Pregnancy Association, at least 60,000 cases of HG are reported by women treated in hospitals. Symptoms include severe nausea and vomiting, inability to hold down any food, decrease in urination, confusion, fainting, rapid heart rate, and other troubling signs. If you experience any of these symptoms, contact your health care professional.

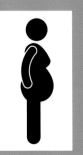

Peppermint Tea

Peppermint is a common remedy for nausea and indigestion. Steep a peppermint tea bag in a mug of hot water for three to five minutes, and drink two to three times a day for relief of morning sickness symptoms. Be aware, however, that if you're suffering from heartburn, peppermint tea may make it worse.

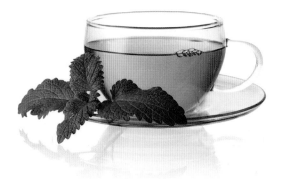

❧ MUSCLE CRAMPS ❧

A muscle cramp is a sudden tightness and pain in your muscle, caused by an involuntary contraction. Muscle cramps are sometimes called charley horses and can have various causes, including excessive exercise (especially in hot weather), fatigue, dehydration, or deficiencies in potassium, magnesium, or calcium. Muscle cramps generally go away on their own, however if the pain is excessive or doesn't improve with home treatment, you may want to see a doctor. Otherwise, there are several home remedies to help relax your muscles and ease your pain.

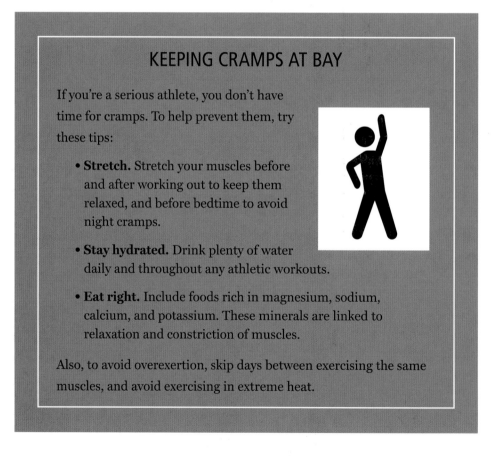

KEEPING CRAMPS AT BAY

If you're a serious athlete, you don't have time for cramps. To help prevent them, try these tips:

- **Stretch.** Stretch your muscles before and after working out to keep them relaxed, and before bedtime to avoid night cramps.

- **Stay hydrated.** Drink plenty of water daily and throughout any athletic workouts.

- **Eat right.** Include foods rich in magnesium, sodium, calcium, and potassium. These minerals are linked to relaxation and constriction of muscles.

Also, to avoid overexertion, skip days between exercising the same muscles, and avoid exercising in extreme heat.

Pickle Juice

While it sounds strange, it's common for athletic trainers to give athletes pickle juice to relieve muscle cramps. Putting this remedy to the test, in a 2010 study at Brigham Young University, researchers gave cramp-stricken athletes water or pickle juice to ease their pain. Surprisingly, the pickle juice offered significantly greater relief than water or simply waiting out the cramp. The theory is that something in the juice—possibly vinegar—may trigger nervous-system receptors that in turn send out signals to stop the spasms. Study participants received 2.5 ounces of pickle juice strained from a jar of dill pickles.

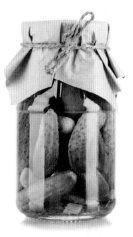

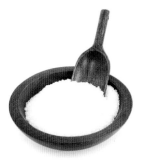

Epsom Salt Bath

Epsom salt is comprised of magnesium, which relaxes muscles and eases pain. For relief of muscle cramps, add 2 cups of Epsom salt to a tub of warm water and soak for fifteen minutes. You can also eat foods rich in magnesium, such as dark leafy greens, nuts, and beans.

Heat

To relax your aching muscle and stimulate blood flow, apply a heating pad or hot washcloth to the affected area. For best results, use heat for twenty minutes on, twenty minutes off. You can also try a warm bath for relief.

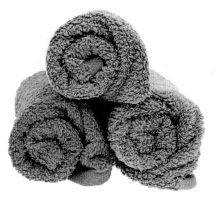

❧ NAIL FUNGUS ❧

Nail fungus is an infection of the toenails or fingernails, characterized by a yellowing and thickening of one or more nails. Like athlete's foot, this condition is caused by fungi often picked up in damp environments such as pools, showers, or locker rooms. In addition to the discoloration and thickness, other symptoms of nail fungus may include brittle and/or dull nails, pain, and a foul smell. While severe cases may require a visit to the doctor and prescription drugs, nail fungus often responds to over-the-counter medications and home care.

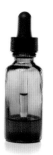

Tee Tree Oil

With its antifungal properties, tea tree oil can be effective in treating nail fungus. Dilute the oil, using a ratio of one part oil to nine parts water, and apply twice a day. Or, you can add 4–5 drops of oil to a shallow tub of water and soak your feet for fifteen minutes.

Clove Oil

Clove oil has natural antifungal and anesthetic properties, due to the presence of eugenol, a chemical compound known to inhibit fungi and dull pain. Combine 2–4 drops of clove oil with a teaspoon of a carrier oil such as olive or coconut oil to dilute it, and apply to the affected area with a cotton ball twice a day.

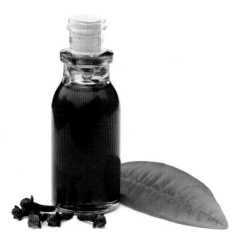

DIABETES AND NAIL FUNGUS

People with diabetes are at greater risk of developing skin and foot problems, including infection. Fungal infections are often more serious in diabetes patients, due to poor circulation and loss of feeling that often leaves them undetected for longer periods of time.

If you have diabetes and notice any symptoms of nail fungus, consult your doctor.

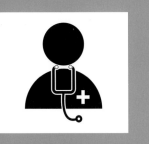

Coconut Oil

The fatty acids in coconut oil make it a potent antifungal. Apply a thin layer of coconut oil to the affected nail two to three times a day.

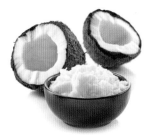

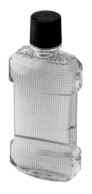

Mouthwash

Mouthwash containing alcohol, such as Listerine, has antimicrobial properties, reducing bacteria and warding off fungal infections. Soak your toenails in mouthwash for fifteen to twenty minutes, twice a day, until you see results. You can also combine the mouthwash with an equal part white vinegar, as the acidity of the vinegar makes it hard for fungi to thrive and spread.

❧ NAUSEA ❧

Nausea is a general term for that queasy, uncomfortable feeling in your stomach, often followed by vomiting. It can have many causes, including gastroenteritis (the "stomach flu"), morning sickness during pregnancy, certain medicines or medical procedures, migraines, overconsumption of alcohol, motion sickness, food poisoning, or even just nerves or jitters. No matter the cause, when you're experiencing nausea, you want it gone—*fast*. For the occasional mild-to-moderate bout of nausea, try one of the following home remedies to get you back on track.

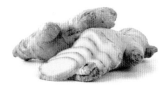

Ginger

Ginger is a popular treatment for nausea, although you'll want to use the real thing, if possible, instead of ginger ale, which often contains too little ginger to be effective. To make ginger tea, combine twelve slices of ginger with 3 cups of water in a pot and simmer for twenty minutes. Remove from heat and strain. Ginger candies are also available if you need relief on the go.

WHEN TO CALL THE DOCTOR

If your nausea is caused by an underlying medical condition—or leads to severe vomiting or other symptoms—you may need medical attention. Seek medical attention if your nausea:

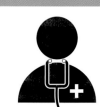

- Lasts for several days

- Is accompanied by fever

- Results in severe vomiting and/or diarrhea

For nausea remedies related to specific conditions, see the entries on *food poisoning, hangovers, headaches,* and *morning sickness.*

Peppermint Tea

Peppermint tea is a common and effective remedy for nausea. To make this tea, add dried peppermint leaves to a mug of boiled water and steep for five to ten minutes. Strain and drink as needed. Consider avoiding peppermint if you suffer from heartburn or reflux, as peppermint may make these conditions worse, and do not give peppermint to an infant or young child.

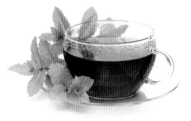

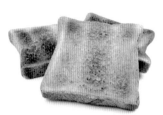

Milk Toast

This folk remedy is a popular nausea treatment. The toast helps to absorb excess stomach acid, while the milk soothes the stomach. Lightly toast a slice of bread and coat with a thin layer of butter. Warm a glass of milk and crumble the bread into the milk. Eat slowly with a spoon for relief.

Lemons

The theory behind using lemons to fight nausea is that the smell triggers the digestive system, stimulating the body to secrete bile and gastric juice, aiding in digestion. Slice a lemon in half and breathe in its powerful aroma to counter your nausea.

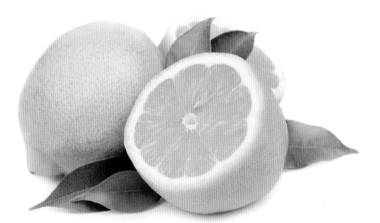

❧ NOSEBLEEDS ❧

While some people rarely get bloody noses, for others—especially children—they are a common nuisance. Most nosebleeds come from the front of the nose (known as *anterior* nosebleeds), and are triggered either by some trauma, such as getting hit in the nose with a ball, or irritation caused by nose picking, frequent nose blowing, or dried-out nasal tissues due to cold, dry weather, typically experienced in winter. In rare cases, bleeding stems from an artery in the back of the nose (a *posterior* nosebleed), which may require emergency care in a hospital. For most nosebleeds, however, home care and an ounce of prevention will do the trick.

Saline

If you're prone to nosebleeds, especially in the winter, keep your nose lubricated with a saline nasal spray or saline nose drops. To make your own saline solution, add ½–1 teaspoon of salt to 1 cup of water. Boil the mixture and allow to cool completely. Use the saline two to three times a day and before going to sleep.

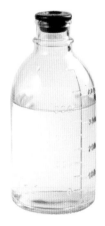

WHEN TO SEEK HELP

Call your doctor if you have more than two nosebleeds a month, if you're on blood thinners, or if you have a medical condition that affects blood clotting. If you can't get your nosebleed to stop or if it's accompanied by rash, fever, dizziness, or trouble breathing, seek emergency medical care.

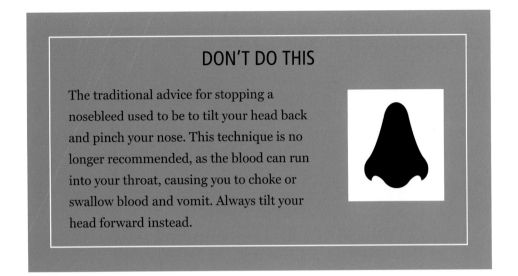

DON'T DO THIS

The traditional advice for stopping a nosebleed used to be to tilt your head back and pinch your nose. This technique is no longer recommended, as the blood can run into your throat, causing you to choke or swallow blood and vomit. Always tilt your head forward instead.

Give It a Pinch

To stop a nosebleed, lean your head forward, and using your thumb and forefinger, pinch your nose where the bones meet the cartilage. Pinch your nose for five minutes; if this doesn't work, try for another five minutes. If your nose is still bleeding, then call a doctor.

Vitamin C

To strengthen capillary walls in your nose and prevent future nosebleeds, take 1,000 milligrams a day of vitamin C.

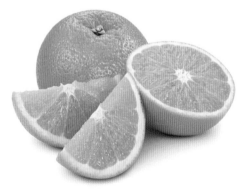

❧ OILY HAIR ❧

You just washed your hair yesterday, but it's already greasy again. What gives? When sebaceous glands in your scalp produce too much sebum—an oily substance that lubricates the hair and skin—your hair appears oily and unwashed. Oily hair can have several causes, including hormone changes during puberty or pregnancy, overuse of styling products, too much brushing, or eating fatty, oily foods. Fortunately, with a few natural fixes, it's possible for your hair to shine—without all that extra oil.

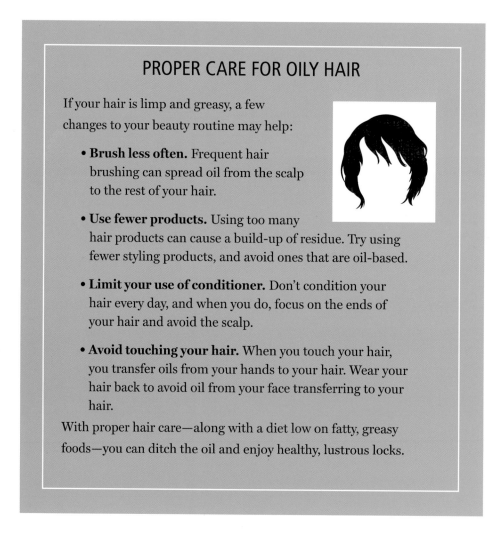

PROPER CARE FOR OILY HAIR

If your hair is limp and greasy, a few changes to your beauty routine may help:

- **Brush less often.** Frequent hair brushing can spread oil from the scalp to the rest of your hair.

- **Use fewer products.** Using too many hair products can cause a build-up of residue. Try using fewer styling products, and avoid ones that are oil-based.

- **Limit your use of conditioner.** Don't condition your hair every day, and when you do, focus on the ends of your hair and avoid the scalp.

- **Avoid touching your hair.** When you touch your hair, you transfer oils from your hands to your hair. Wear your hair back to avoid oil from your face transferring to your hair.

With proper hair care—along with a diet low on fatty, greasy foods—you can ditch the oil and enjoy healthy, lustrous locks.

Lemon Juice

A natural astringent, lemon juice removes excess oil and restores your scalp's pH balance. Mix ¼ cup lemon juice in 2 cups of water, and massage into your scalp and hair. After a few minutes, rinse the mixture from your hair. Follow these steps two to three times a week.

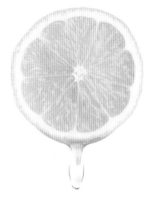

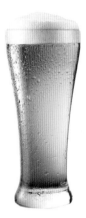

Beer

While it may sound odd, beer actually makes for a healthy hair rinse for oily hair sufferers. The alcohol is drying, and the malt and hops contain proteins that can repair hair and give it volume. Use a can or bottle of warm, flat beer as a rinse after shampooing. Leave the beer in for a few minutes and then rinse.

Apple Cider Vinegar

Apple cider vinegar acts as an astringent, helping to dry up excess oil, and balances your scalp's pH level, reducing the overproduction of oil. Add 2 tablespoons of apple cider vinegar to 1 cup of water and wash your hair with the mixture. Leave on for a few minutes before rinsing.

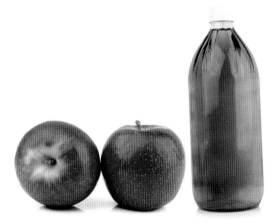

❧ OILY SKIN ❧

While everyone wants a healthy glow, shiny skin can be unattractive and lead to acne and blackheads. Oily skin is caused by the sebaceous glands in the skin producing too much sebum, an oily, waxy substance that protects the skin and hair. Factors contributing to oily skin can include heredity, hormonal changes related to pregnancy or birth control pills, or a diet rich in oily, fatty foods. While many over-the-counter products address oily skin, a number of household items found right in your kitchen also work to remove excess oil.

Yogurt

Yogurt contains lactic acid, which can slow down sebum production in the skin. Apply a thin layer of plain yogurt over your entire face and leave on for ten to fifteen minutes. Rinse off with cool water. Repeat this process daily.

Lemon Juice

Lemon juice is a natural astringent that exfoliates the skin. Dilute the juice of one lemon with an equal amount of water and apply the mixture to your face. Once the juice dries, rinse it off with cool water and apply an oil-free moisturizer to prevent the juice from drying out your skin. Do this several times a week.

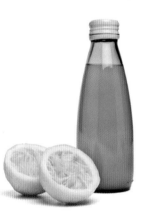

Sea Salt

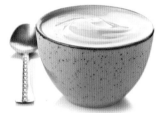

The drying power of salt can exfoliate and remove excess oil from your skin. Add 1 teaspoon of salt to 2 cups of water and mix. Use a spray bottle to mist the mixture over your face, without rinsing. You can do this every day if needed to keep your skin oil-free.

Tomato Juice

Another natural astringent, tomatoes tighten pores and contain acids that absorb oil. Place a diced tomato in a grinder or blender until you get a thick paste. Apply a thin layer to your skin. Once it dries, rinse off with cool water and apply an oil-free moisturizer. Follow this routine twice a week.

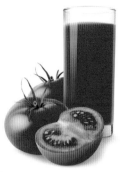

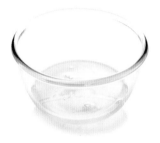

Egg Whites

Egg whites can shrink your pores, allowing less oil onto your face. Separate the egg white from one egg; pour it in a bowl, add a few drops of lemon juice, and whisk. Apply the mixture to your face and allow it to harden into a mask, for about fifteen minutes. Wash the mask off with warm water and apply an oil-free moisturizer. Repeat once or twice a week.

RICE PAPER

If you're out and about, heading to an important meeting, or in the midst of humidity wave, you may need to take care of oily skin on the go. For these occasions, you can purchase rice-paper blotting tissue from any beauty supply store. They come in small packages, about the size of a credit card, and can be used to wipe away the oil. Often they are coated with a light powder, so be sure to match your skin tone if you're purchasing that variety.

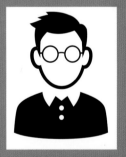

If your oily skin is causing breakouts, see the chapter in this book about *acne* for more treatments.

❧ POISON IVY AND POISON OAK ❧

If you've been camping, you're probably familiar with the perils of poison ivy and poison oak. These plants, which are recognizable by their distinctive leaves—each made up of three small leaflets—contain an oil called urushiol, which causes an itchy rash when it comes into contact with your skin. While it's best to avoid any contact with these plants, should you unexpectedly encounter them, symptoms may include red, itchy skin, hives, and blisters. It can take a few days for the rash to appear, and it may last two to three weeks. While uncomfortable, most cases of poison ivy or poison oak rash aren't serious and can be treated at home.

WHEN TO SEEK HELP

According to the American Academy of Dermatology, you should seek immediate medical attention if, after coming into contact with poison ivy or poison oak, you experience trouble breathing or swallowing, have multiple rashes or a rash that covers much of your body, your eyelids swell shut, or the rash is on your face or genitals. Also see a doctor if the rash doesn't improve after a few weeks.

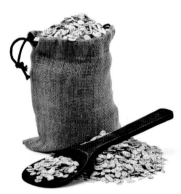

Oatmeal

To relieve the itch, bathe in colloidal (or finely ground) oatmeal. Colloidal oatmeal is available at drugstores, or you can make your own by placing 2 cups of oatmeal in a blender, and blending until it forms a fine powder. Sprinkle the oatmeal in lukewarm bathwater and soak for ten to fifteen minutes. Alternatively, you can apply regular oatmeal, while still warm, to the affected area as a paste.

ACT QUICKLY

If you've gotten the oil from a poison ivy or oak plant on your skin, immediately wash it off with soap and water. While there's no guarantee you won't get a rash, if you act quickly, you may be able to avoid it.

Calamine Lotion

This is the traditional remedy for poison ivy or oak rash, and is available at drugstores. Apply a small amount to the affected area as needed to relieve itching.

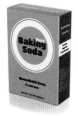

Baking Soda

Baking soda is known to relieve itching. Sprinkle ½ cup in your bath, or mix 1 teaspoon of baking soda in 4 ounces of water and apply the mixture directly to the affected area.

Aloe Vera

Aloe vera's anti-inflammatory, antimicrobial properties can relieve swelling and itchiness. Apply fresh gel from an aloe vera plant directly to the affected area. The plant is preferable to over-the-counter gels, which aren't as effective.

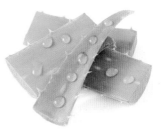

❧ PSORIASIS ❧

Psoriasis is a chronic skin condition characterized by thick, red, scaly patches, typically on the outside of the elbows, knees, and scalp—although they can appear on any part of the body. The patches may itch or burn, and symptoms tend to go through stages of worsening and then improving. Experts link psoriasis to an immune disorder that causes an overproduction of skin cells. Psoriasis may be genetic or triggered by environmental factors, ranging from cold weather to obesity to various infections. While there is no cure for psoriasis, doctors typically treat symptoms with topical creams and/or oral medications. To calm the itching and scaling of psoriasis, you also may wish to try these alternative remedies.

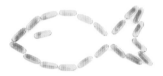

Fish Oil

Omega-3 fatty acids found in certain fish, such as sardines, tuna, and mackerel, may reduce the inflammation associated with psoriasis. Add two servings of fish a week to your diet, or add fish oil capsules to your supplement regimen. Recommended dosages vary widely, so consult a doctor on the appropriate of amount of DHA and EPA for you.

NOT JUST SKIN DEEP

According to the National Psoriasis Foundation, people with psoriasis have an elevated risk of developing other medical conditions, such as arthritis, cardiovascular disease, diabetes, and depression. If you have symptoms of psoriasis, be sure to speak to your doctor, so that she can monitor you for these and other health risks.

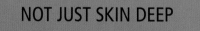

Apple Cider Vinegar

If psoriasis is causing scalp itch, anti-inflammatory apple cider vinegar may offer relief. Dilute the vinegar, using thee parts water to one part ACV, and apply directly to your scalp a few times a week. Avoid this remedy, however, if the skin on your scalp is cracked or bleeding.

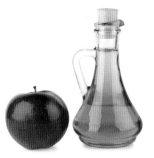

Salt

Taking a warm bath containing Dead Sea salts or Epsom salts may relieve your itching and remove scales. Soak for fifteen minutes and apply moisturizer immediately afterward. Make sure the water isn't too hot, or you might exacerbate your symptoms.

Aloe Vera

The gel of the aloe vera plant may ease the itching and inflammation of psoriasis. Cut open a leaf, squeeze out the gel, and apply it directly to the affected area. Repeat several times a day until you experience some relief.

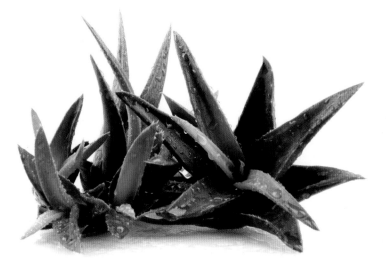

❧ RASHES ❧

A rash refers to irritation of the skin. The affected area may be itchy, red, swollen, or covered in blisters. Rashes can be caused by many things, from allergies to eczema to contact with poison ivy. A common rash is contact dermatitis, which simply means that your skin has come into contact with an irritant—such as detergent, soap, makeup, or certain chemicals—that has caused you to develop a red, itchy rash where the contact occurred. While these rashes are generally not dangerous, and tend to resolve on their own within a few weeks, they can be extremely uncomfortable and, should you repeatedly scratch the area and break the skin, can potentially become infected. Fortunately, there are simple home remedies that can reduce the itching and help your skin to heal.

Oatmeal

To calm itchy skin, bathe in colloidal (finely ground) oatmeal. You can make your own by placing 2 cups of oatmeal in a blender, and blending until it forms a fine powder. Sprinkle the oatmeal in lukewarm bathwater and soak for ten to fifteen minutes. Alternatively, you can apply regular oatmeal, once it's cooled, to the rash area as a paste.

FOR MORE IDEAS

To learn more about specific types of rashes and their remedies, see the chapters in this book on *allergies, chickenpox, diaper rash, eczema, hives, poison ivy* and *poison oak, psoriasis, ringworm,* and *rosacea.*

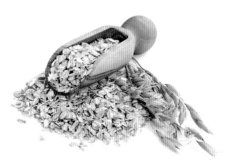

Basil

Basil leaves contain pain-numbing eugenol, as well as camphor and thymol, substances that soothe itchy skin. Rub crushed fresh basil leaves directly on the skin for relief.

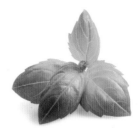

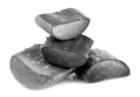

Aloe Vera

With its moisturizing, anti-inflammatory properties, aloe vera can relieve itchy, swollen skin. Apply fresh gel from an aloe vera plant directly to the affected area. The plant is preferable to over-the-counter gels, which may contain alcohol that can dry the skin.

HEAT RASH

It's mid-July, and your skin is prickly and covered in red bumps. Heat rash occurs when sweat glands become blocked; unable to evaporate from your skin, the trapped sweat causes inflammation. To treat heat rash, try the following:

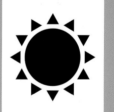

- **Ice:** Cooling the skin can stop heat rash in its tracks. Wrap ice in cloth and apply it to your skin for five to ten minutes at a time.

- **Baking soda:** Baking soda can relieve itching. Place $1/2$–1 cup baking soda in slightly cool water and soak for fifteen to twenty minutes.

- **Baby powder:** Dust baby or talcum powder on your skin to absorb extra moisture.

To avoid heat rash, wear lightweight, loose-fitting clothing; use air conditioning when it's hot; and drink plenty of water.

❧ RAZOR BURN ❧

You may enjoy the look and feel of a smooth, clean shave—but there's nothing attractive about the red, angry-looking rash that sometimes accompanies it. True to its name, razor burn may burn or itch, and can appear wherever you shave. Razor burn may be caused by shaving with a dull blade, which requires you to press harder and cuts unevenly, or by shaving dry or sensitive skin. Razor burn generally fades with time, but if you want that rash gone quickly, try these easy remedies for relief.

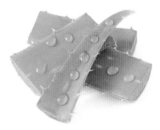

Aloe Vera

Aloe vera gel is moisturizing and anti-inflammatory; in addition, its antimicrobial properties can help prevent broken skin from getting infected. Apply fresh gel from an aloe vera plant directly to the affected area. Use the plant if possible, instead of over-the-counter gels, which may contain alcohol that can dry and further irritate the skin.

Tea Bags

The tannins in black tea reduce inflammation and redness. To try this remedy, press two to three cool, wet tea bags on the affected area for several minutes.

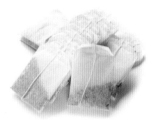

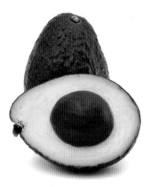

Avocado

Full of healthy fats and vitamins A, D, and E, avocados can reduce inflammation and cool irritated skin. Mash up a fresh avocado and apply directly to red, itchy areas to soothe them.

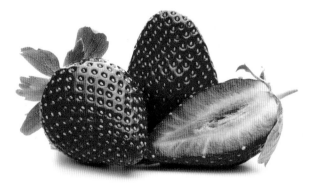

Strawberries

Strawberries not only smell great, but they can reduce swelling and redness of the skin. Mash up a few strawberries and mix in some sour cream, in order to make a paste. Apply the paste to the razor burn and leave on for ten to fifteen minutes before washing it off with warm water.

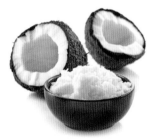

Coconut Oil

With its hydrating and anti-inflammatory properties, coconut oil can take the sting out of razor burn and help to heal irritated skin. Apply the oil directly to the affected area.

RASH OR INGROWN HAIR?

Bumps that appear on your skin after shaving may be ingrown hairs, which occur when hair curls back into the skin instead of growing out of it. Ingrown hairs may look like pimples, and are often accompanied by irritation, pain, and inflammation. See the chapter on *ingrown hairs* for more information.

❧ RINGWORM ❧

Ringworm is a skin infection caused by a fungus called tinea. While it's common in children, anyone can get ringworm, and it's easily passed on in warm, moist areas such as pools and locker rooms. You can also contract ringworm by sharing contaminated objects, such as hairbrushes or clothing, or from infected pets. Symptoms of ringworm include raised patches on the skin that are often redder around the edges, with clear centers, causing a ring-like appearance. The patches may itch or form blisters, and can affect various parts of the body. When they appear on the feet, they are known as athlete's foot; on the groin, jock itch. Various over-the-counter antifungal medications are available to treat ringworm; however, if the infection is on your scalp or doesn't respond to home care, your doctor may prescribe oral medication. To relieve the itching and discomfort of ringworm, try the following natural remedies.

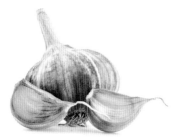

Garlic

Garlic has antifungal and antibacterial properties, and is used for many types of infections. Peel and crush a clove of garlic, and apply it to the affected area, securing it with a bandage overnight.

RINGWORM: NOT JUST FOR HUMANS

It's possible for pets such as dogs and cats to catch ringworm—from people and from other animals—and to pass it along as well. Therefore, it's important to take your pet to the vet if it's showing any signs of this condition. Be sure to thoroughly wash your hands with soap and water after handling an animal you believe may have ringworm.

Tea Tree Oil

Tea tree oil is active against many fungi and bacteria. Create a mixture of 50 percent tea tree oil and 50 percent olive oil, and rub the combination on the affected area twice a day.

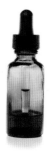

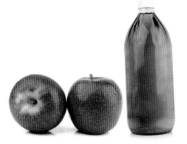

Apple Cider Vinegar

With its antifungal and anti-inflammatory properties, apple cider vinegar is a natural remedy for ringworm. It also balances your skin's pH level, making it less hospitable to fungi and bacteria. Use a cotton ball to apply undiluted vinegar directly to the rash three to five times a day, for at least three days.

Lavender Oil

Lavender oil has antifungal properties and mild sedative powers, to both relieve symptoms and fight the ringworm infection. Apply a few drops of oil directly on the affected area several times a day.

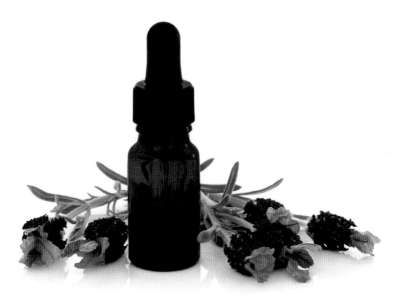

❧ ROSACEA ❧

It can be hard to face the world when you have rosacea. This chronic skin condition affects the face, causing persistent redness, small red or pus-filled bumps resembling acne, visible blood vessels, raised red patches, and even swelling of the nose or redness of the eyes. Rosacea is more common in women and tends to begin after age thirty, with fair-skinned people who easily blush or flush most vulnerable to developing this condition. Symptoms tend to come and go, and worsen with age. No one knows what causes rosacea; it may be genetic, with flare-ups triggered by environment factors such as exposure to sun, stress, hot weather, and alcohol consumption. While there is no treatment, doctors sometimes manage symptoms with antibiotics with anti-inflammatory effects or with acne medication. To get your rosacea flare-ups under control, you can also try some home remedies and lifestyle changes.

Green Tea

Green tea has anti-inflammatory and antioxidant properties, and also can help to protect the skin from harmful rays of the sun. Certain face creams contain green tea extract, or you can cool a batch of green tea in the fridge, and apply it to your face with a washcloth for twenty minutes when you have an outbreak.

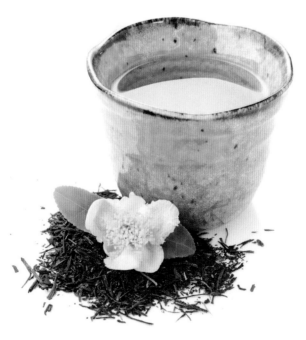

Probiotics

Recent research has shown that probiotics, applied topically or taken orally, can benefit rosacea sufferers. Used topically, the "good" bacteria found in probiotics can distract the immune system from responding to the "bad" bacteria found naturally on the skin, avoiding an inflammatory immune response. Internally, probiotics can interfere with inflammation that results when stress and poor diet slow digestion, causing the gut to be overrun with bad bacteria that eventually "leak" into the bloodstream. To benefit from probiotics, you can use an over-the-counter probiotic mask, cream, or cleanser—or you can add probiotics to your diet (in the form of kefir or yogurts containing "live active cultures") or take a probiotic supplement.

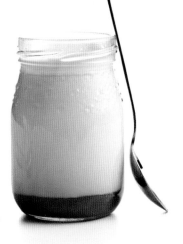

PUT ON A GOOD FACE

The easiest way to treat a rosacea flare-up is to avoid getting one. Avoid common triggers by:

- Always using sunscreen, with an SPF of 30 or higher

- Avoiding alcohol

- Steering clear of spicy foods, and consuming hot foods and beverages in moderation

- Avoiding hot baths, hot tubs, and saunas

In addition, stress can be a trigger—and, unfortunately, a rosacea flare-up on your face can add to your stress. Therefore, if you have rosacea, it's important to have a support network, talk to your doctor, and get the help you need.

⌁ SCARS ⌁

After you've healed from an injury, the last thing you want is a permanent memory of it. Yet that's what a scar is—new skin that grows over a healed cut, burn, incision, or other wound. Often this skin is a slightly different color and thickness than the surrounding skin. Scars fade over time but, depending on the scar, this process can take months or years—and the scar never really goes away. The degree of the scar depends on factors including the location of the injury, your age, and the severity of the wound. While scarring is a natural part of the skin's healing process, more prominent scars can be damaging to a person's self-esteem. Dermatologists offer various procedures to treat scars, including laser surgery, steroid injections, dermabrasion, and more. At home, you can try natural alternatives to reduce the appearance of scars.

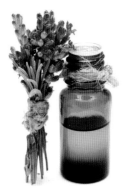

Lavender Oil

Lavender oil aids in healing and cell regeneration, which may prevent and treat scars. Clean new wounds with water containing 4–5 drops of lavender oil to accelerate healing. For existing scars, apply 2–4 drops of lavender oil to the affected area several times a day.

Coconut Oil

Coconut oil stimulates production and replacement of collagen, helping the body to reabsorb the thicker collagen formed during scarring and generate new, natural collagen. Gently rub warmed coconut oil directly on the scar several times a day.

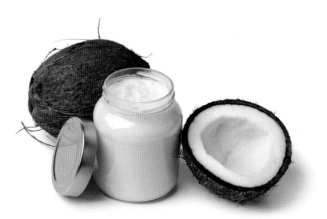

SCAR PREVENTION

How quickly and effectively a wound heals can determine whether or not there will be a scar—and how severe it will be. To prevent a scar, try the following:

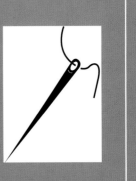

- **Cover a cut.** Use an antibiotic ointment and keep the cut covered to avoid an infection that can delay healing and lead to greater scarring.

- **Consider stitches.** For wide, gaping cuts, visit an emergency room to see if you need stitches. Stitches make for a smaller wound area, requiring collagen to seal it.

- **Keep scars out of sunlight.** UV rays from the sun cause inflammation and other effects that prevent the formation of new collagen. Keep the scar covered or use sunscreen with a minimum SPF of 30.

While sometimes scarring is inevitable, by properly treating a wound, you can reduce your chances of having a long-lasting, unsightly reminder of your injury.

Aloe Vera

Aloe vera gel softens skin, reduces inflammation, and stimulates collagen production. Apply the gel of an aloe vera plant to the scar several times a day.

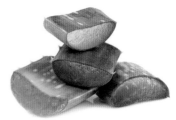

❧ SHIN SPLINTS ❧

Shin splints are the bane of runners and athletes everywhere who try to push themselves to the next level a little too quickly. Also known as medial tibial stress syndrome, shin splints cause pain along the shinbone, the bone in the front of your lower leg. This condition is generally caused by overexerting the muscles around the shinbone, often as a result of changing your exercise routine, running longer distances than usual, or wearing worn-out or improper footwear while working out. Fortunately, shin splints usually aren't serious, and with a little rest and home care, you'll be back on your feet once more.

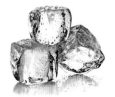

Ice
To calm those inflamed muscles around your shinbone, apply ice to the affected area. Wrap the ice in a thin cloth and apply to your skin for twenty minutes at a time, a few times a day.

PREVENTING SHIN SPLINTS

Though shin splints are incredibly common, that doesn't mean they aren't preventable. There are several things you can do to cut this pain in the shins out of your life:

- Wear supportive, quality shoes.

- Warm up slowly before a hard workout.

- Work to make sure the supportive muscles in your ankles and hips are in good shape.

- Stretch your legs thoroughly after your workout.

- Stop working out the moment you feel pain.

Practice these precautions regularly and not only will your shin splints go away, but you'll improve your overall health and fitness.

Rest

The best thing you can do for shin splints is to take a break from the activity that caused the problem in the first place. Take two to four weeks off from running or other high-impact exercises; you can walk or engage in low-impact activities such as swimming, but don't push yourself beyond that until you're healed. When you do return to your previous routine, start slow and make sure to stretch before and after exercising.

WHEN TO GET HELP

Call the doctor if self-care doesn't ease your pain after a few weeks, or if your shin becomes red or warm to the touch.

Stretches

There are various stretches recommended for people suffering from shin splints. One such stretch, recommended by *Runner's World*, involves kneeling on the floor with your legs and feet together, and then slowly sitting back on your calves and heels. If you're doing it right, you begin to feel tension in the muscles around your shin. Hold for ten to twelve seconds before relaxing your muscles, and then repeat.

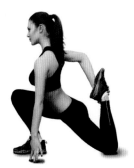

Vitamin D

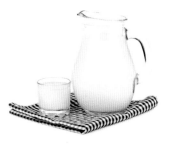

Vitamin D is essential for building strong bones and muscles. If you frequently place stress on your shins, consider adding vitamin D to your diet, by including fortified milk, eggs, and fatty fish. If you're taking a supplement, according to the National Institutes of Health, the recommended daily allowance of vitamin D is 600 IU.

❧ SINUSITIS ❧

Sinusitis occurs when the tissue lining the sinuses becomes swollen, causing mucus to build up—making breathing difficult and placing you at risk for bacterial and fungal infections. Other symptoms may include facial swelling and pain, headaches, yellow or green discharge from the nose, fever, and cough. Sinusitis may be acute or chronic. Acute sinusitis is commonly caused by colds, allergies, or infections, and usually resolves within four weeks. If symptoms persist longer than twelve weeks, you may have chronic sinusitis. Doctors often treat acute sinusitis with over-the-counter decongestants or, in cases of bacterial infection, antibiotics. People who suffer from chronic sinusitis may benefit from vaporizers, saline drops, short-term use of decongestants, or oral steroids to reduce inflammation. In more severe cases, doctors may recommend surgical options. To manage the symptoms of sinusitis, you also may wish to try to the alternative treatments listed below.

Turmeric and Ginger Root

Turmeric is yellow spice commonly used in Indian cuisine. Its active compound, curcumin, may reduce inflammation in the body. Ginger also has anti-inflammatory and decongestant properties. Make a soothing tea by adding ½ cup each of turmeric and ginger to 2 cups of boiling water. Reduce to a simmer for ten minutes and then strain.

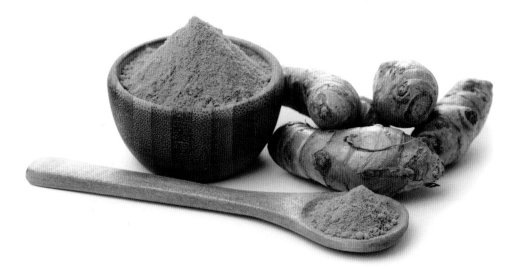

Grapefruit Seed Extract

Made from the seeds and pulp of grapefruits, this extract is a natural antibiotic and antioxidant that relieves inflammation and can help clear out the sinuses. You can find grapefruit seed extract at most health food stores. Add a few drops of the extract to a glass of warm water. You can add a quarter teaspoon of salt for extra mucus-thinning power. Irrigate your nose with this solution using a neti pot or nasal bulb syringe.

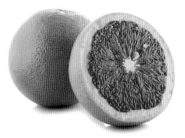

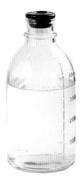

Saline

Saline washes can help to thin mucus and flush it from your nasal passages. To make your own saline solution, add ½–1 teaspoon of salt to 1 cup of water. Boil the mixture and allow to cool completely. You can use a nasal bulb syringe or neti pot daily to pour the solution into your nostril.

WHEN TO CALL THE DOCTOR

Call your doctor immediately if you have other troubling symptoms such as:

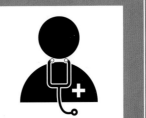

- Fever

- Severe headache

- Shortness of breath

- Changes in your vision

And if your sinusitis lasts longer than two weeks, contact your physician.

❦ SKIN TAGS ❦

A skin tag is a small, harmless growth on the skin that may be flesh-colored or slightly darker, and may be attached to the skin by a stalk, or peduncle. They typically occur in areas where skin rubs against skin, such as the eyelids, armpits, or neck, although they can grow anywhere. Certain people are more likely to develop skin tags than others, either because of genetics, obesity, or other factors including pregnancy and diabetes. Skin tags are generally painless; however, if you're bothered by the appearance of a skin tag, or if it's in a location where it rubs against clothing or skin, causing irritation, you may wish to remove it. A doctor can do this with surgery, or by freezing or burning off the skin tag. Should you wish to avoid these methods, you can try a few basic home treatments that may remove the skin tag without a painful procedure.

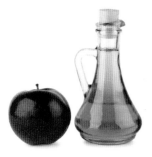

Apple Cider Vinegar

The acidic nature of the vinegar can cause the skin tag to fall off naturally. Wash the area with soap and water and dry completely. Use a cotton swab to apply ACV directly on the skin tag, and hold it there for a minute or two. Do this daily until the skin tag turns dark and then falls off.

Lemon Juice

The citric acid in lemon juice can help to break down excess cells and dry out skin tags. Clean and dry the area around the skin tag. Squeeze fresh lemon juice onto a cotton ball and apply it to the skin tag three times a day.

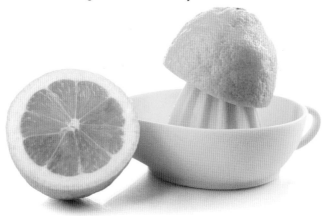

DON'T TRY THIS AT HOME!

While it may be tempting to cut off a skin tag, don't do it! Here are five very good reasons not to:

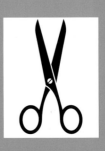

- It might not be a skin tag, as other serious conditions look a lot like skin tags.

- You can cause a fair amount of bleeding and leave the area vulnerable to infection.

- Some larger tags require anesthesia for removal because the procedure can cause severe pain.

- It's rare, but the appearance of skin tags may indicate an endocrine or hormonal syndrome.

- Treatment can vary depending on the size and location, so a scissor snip approach can cause more harm than good.

If you're really concerned, and home remedies aren't working, consult your doctor.

Tea Tree Oil

A natural astringent, tea tree oil is used for many skin ailments and is a popular home treatment for skin tags. First clean and dry the affected area. Then add a few drops of tea tree oil to a water-soaked cotton ball and rub it on the skin tag several times a day until it dries up and falls off.

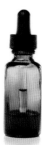

❧ SNORING ❧

According to the American Academy of Otolaryngology—Head and Neck Surgery, a whopping 45 percent of normal adults snore, while 25 percent are habitual snorers. That's a lot of nighttime racket! Snoring is the result of breathing being blocked while you sleep; tissues in your airway strike one another and vibrate, making the all-too-familiar snoring sound. Anyone can snore; however, men tend to do so more. In addition, being overweight, consuming alcohol, and congestion can contribute to snoring. If snoring is bothering you or (more likely) your partner, you may want to try some simple remedies to help everyone get a good night's sleep.

Steam

Dry air can contribute to congestion, as can mucus from a cold or allergies—all of which can contribute to snoring. Use a vaporizer or humidifier while you sleep to keep the membranes in your nasal passages moist and thin mucus that may be obstructing your breathing. Add a few drops of eucalyptus oil to help clear up congestion.

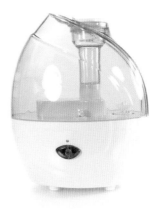

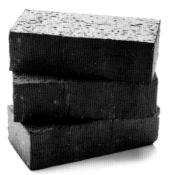

Raised Bed Head

Try elevating the head of your bed to open up your airways while you sleep. Place boards or bricks under the legs of the head of the bed to raise it 4–6 inches. Don't raise the bed more than that, or you may actually end up constricting the airways instead.

Tennis Ball

It may sound strange, but this old trick works for some people whose snoring is related to their sleeping position. Sleeping on your side may reduce snoring; by sewing or taping a tennis ball onto the back of your pajama top, it becomes uncomfortable to sleep on your back, causing you to stay on your side. While not necessarily a long-term solution for chronic snorers or those with sleep apnea, it may provide relief for occasional bouts of snoring.

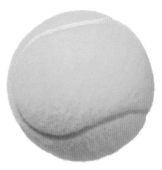

SLEEP APNEA

While snoring is often harmless, it may be a sign of something more serious, such as sleep apnea. With this disorder, breathing can become shallow or even stop for seconds or minutes at a time during sleep. This can cause daytime drowsiness and fatigue, and place you at a higher risk for automobile and workplace accidents. If you don't feel rested after a full night's sleep, or wake up gasping for air, you should consult a doctor.

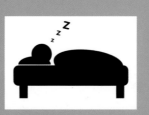

❧ SORE THROAT ❧

Also known as pharyngitis, a sore throat is characterized by a scratchy or painful sensation at the back of the throat, sometimes making it difficult to swallow. A sore throat may be caused by a viral infection, such as a cold or flu; a bacterial infection, such as strep throat; allergies, or other medical conditions. Sore throats generally go away on their own; however, if your sore throat doesn't subside in a few days, or if you have a fever, swollen lymph nodes, white spots on your tonsils, or extreme pain upon swallowing, your doctor may test you for a bacterial infection and possibly prescribe antibiotics. While you're waiting for your sore throat or medicine to run its course, try these home remedies for some quick relief.

IF YOUR CHILD HAS A SORE THROAT

While your child's sore throat is most likely the result of a cold, it can still be concerning. The American Academy of Pediatrics recommends giving children over one year of age warm chicken broth or other warm fluids. Children over six can suck on a hard candy, and kids older than eight can gargle with salt water. Call your child's pediatrician if the sore throat is the only symptom and lasts more than forty-eight hours, if a sore throat with a cold lasts more than five days, or if a fever lasts more than three days. And call the doctor right away if the sore throat is accompanied by a rash, a high fever, difficulty breathing, or other troubling symptoms.

Salt

If your mom made you gargle with saltwater when you had a sore throat as a child, she was on to something. Salt can draw excess fluid out of inflamed tissues, reducing swelling in the throat and making the area less hospitable to bacteria. Dissolve ¼–½ teaspoon of salt in an 8-ounce glass of warm water and briefly gargle several times a day to soothe your irritated throat.

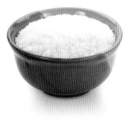

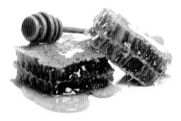

Honey

Honey can soothe and coat your irritated throat, and has natural anti-inflammatory and antibiotic properties. Take 1 tablespoon of organic, raw honey several times a day. (However, never give honey to a child under two years of age.)

Licorice Root

With its antiviral and anti-inflammatory properties, licorice root can be an effective way to ease an irritated throat. Boil ¼ cup licorice root in water to make a tea (add a little ginger for extra soothing power) or add a couple of pinches of licorice powder to your favorite tea for sore throat relief.

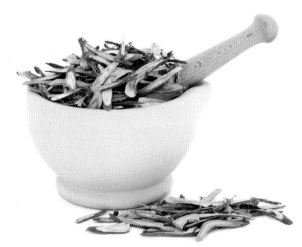

SPRAINS

You land hard after a jump shot and feel a sharp pain in your ankle. You may be experiencing a sprain—an injury to a ligament, or the tissue that connects bones and supports the joints. When you tear or stretch a ligament, pain, swelling, stiffness, and bruising can occur. According to the American Academy of Orthopaedic Surgeons, a sprain is caused by a trauma, such as a fall, that displaces a joint and stretches or possibly tears the supporting ligament. Basic first aid can help mild sprains; more serious sprains should be evaluated by a doctor, who may recommend crutches, physical therapy, or even surgery. To treat a mild sprain, or ease your discomfort as you're healing from a more severe one, try these techniques.

Rice

More than just a popular grain product, RICE is an acronym for a common treatment method for sprains. It stands for:

- **Rest.** For the first twenty-four to forty-eight hours, use the injured body part as little as possible. Use a splint or crutches if necessary.
- **Ice.** To reduce inflammation, use ice wrapped in a thin cloth or a bag of frozen vegetables. Apply to the injury for fifteen to twenty minutes at a time (no longer than that) three to four times a day for the first forty-eight hours after the sprain.
- **Compression.** Use an elastic wrap to snugly wrap the area, making sure not to cut off circulation.
- **Elevation.** Keep the sprain elevated above your heart when possible to reduce swelling.

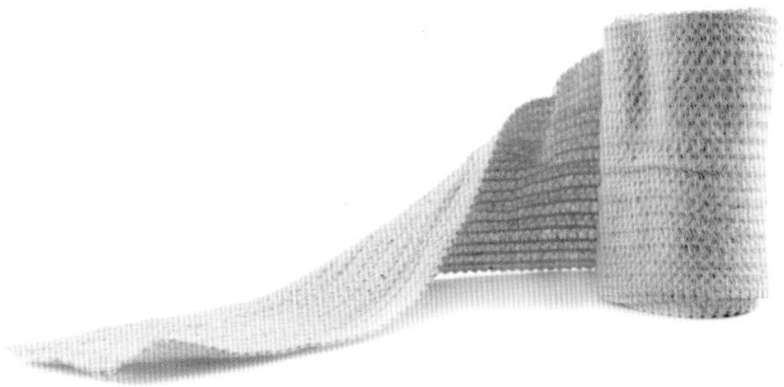

Turmeric

This yellow spice and its active compound, curcumin, reduce inflammation and ease pain. Mix 2–3 tablespoons of turmeric powder with enough water to make a paste. Apply the paste to the sprain, wrap with a bandage, and leave on overnight.

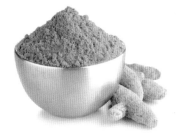

Arnica

Arnica is a plant known for its pain-relieving and anti-inflammatory properties. You can purchase arnica in various forms at health food stores. Massage the arnica onto the sprain for pain relief—but only on *unbroken* skin. Arnica may be toxic if taken internally.

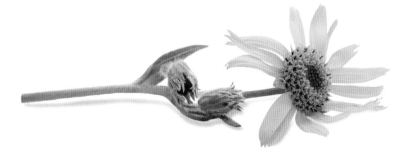

DON'T WAIT

While mild sprains will generally heal within a couple of weeks, severe sprains need to be treated right away to avoid long-term damage. Get medical help immediately if the joint is unusable or numb; you have signs of an infection, such as warm, red skin or a fever; or you think you have a broken bone.

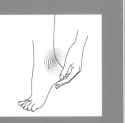

❧ STIES ❧

A sty is a painful infection near the base of the eyelashes, often caused by bacteria. A red lump resembling a pimple forms, which is sometimes filled with pus. The lump will often swell over the course of the infection, before draining after a few days. Anything that brings bacteria in contact with your eyes can place you at risk for sties, including rubbing your eyes, not washing your hands before putting in contact lenses, or using contaminated eye makeup. Sties generally go away on their own, although antibiotics may be necessary for more severe or persistent cases. To relieve the pain of a sty, try these soothing home remedies.

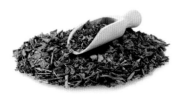

Green Tea

Green tea has natural anti-inflammatory properties that can reduce the swelling and pain of a sty. Soak a green tea bag in warm water and then hold it against the sty for five to ten minutes, several times a day.

Turmeric

The yellow spice turmeric contains the compound curcumin, which naturally reduces inflammation and can relieve the pain of a sty. Add a teaspoon of turmeric to 2 cups of water and boil. Strain and cool, and use the remaining solution to wash the eye. Do this three times a day over the course of several days.

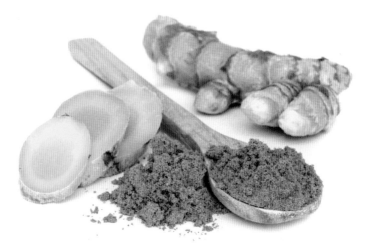

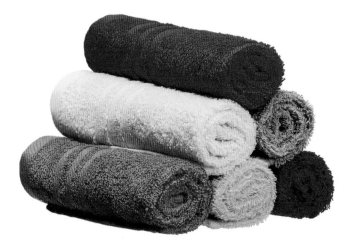

Warm Compress

To relieve the pressure of a sty, you want it to burst and drain. You can often accomplish this by applying a warm washcloth directly to the sty. Leave it on for ten minutes several times a day.

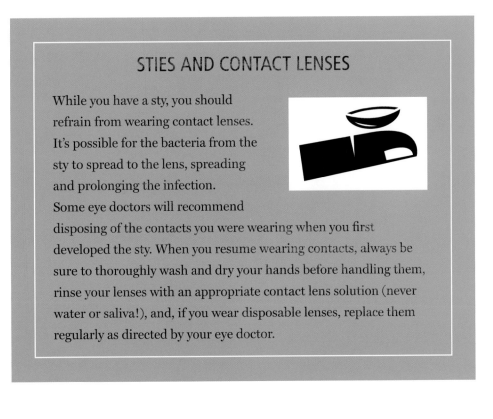

STIES AND CONTACT LENSES

While you have a sty, you should refrain from wearing contact lenses. It's possible for the bacteria from the sty to spread to the lens, spreading and prolonging the infection. Some eye doctors will recommend disposing of the contacts you were wearing when you first developed the sty. When you resume wearing contacts, always be sure to thoroughly wash and dry your hands before handling them, rinse your lenses with an appropriate contact lens solution (never water or saliva!), and, if you wear disposable lenses, replace them regularly as directed by your eye doctor.

❧ SUNBURN ❧

There's nothing like a day at the beach—unless it's followed by days of pain, peeling, and blisters. When you've spent too much time in the sun, exposure to ultraviolet rays can turn your skin red and painful to the touch. With more severe sunburns, you may develop skin blisters, chills, nausea, and even a fever. After a few days, the burn will begin to fade, and you may experience itching as your skin peels—your body's way of shedding the sun-damaged skin. While you should call your doctor if you notice any signs of infection—or if a sunburn is widespread or accompanied by other symptoms such as a high fever, headaches, or confusion—most sunburns can be treated at home. To ease the aftermath of an overly sun-filled day, try these soothing home remedies.

TOO MUCH FUN IN THE SUN

Repeated exposure to ultraviolet rays can prematurely age your skin and place you at risk for skin cancer. To protect your skin, follow these steps:

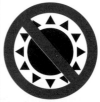

- **Apply sunscreen.** Cover exposed skin with a broad-spectrum sunscreen with a minimum SPF of 30. Apply it liberally thirty minutes before going into the sun, and reapply every couple of hours or after swimming.

- **Dress up.** Wear long sleeves and pants when possible. It can be difficult to apply sunscreen to your scalp, so protect it with a broad-brimmed hat. Wear sunglasses to protect your eyes from the damaging effects of UV light.

- **Time it right.** Avoid the sun between 10 a.m. and 4 p.m., when it's at its strongest.

And remember, just because it's cloudy or overcast, doesn't mean you're not in danger of UV light exposure. Always protect yourself when in the sun—your skin will thank you.

Milk

Got milk? According to The Skin Cancer Foundation, used topically this beverage can cool the skin and create a soothing protein film to ease the discomfort of a sunburn. Soak a washcloth in cold skim milk and apply it directly to the skin for ten minutes at a time.

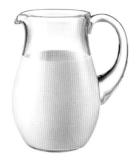

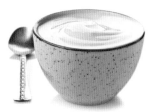

Yogurt

Yogurt can cool a burn, and its probiotics can ease inflammation and help skin heal. Spread a small amount of plain, unsweetened yogurt on the affected area and leave on for five minutes before rinsing it off.

Aloe Vera

A traditional go-to remedy for sunburns, aloe vera gel naturally cools and moisturizes the skin. It also dulls pain, taking the sting out of a sunburn. Scoop the gel from a fresh aloe leaf and apply it directly to the burn. If you don't have an aloe vera plant, you can use store-bought gel, but even ones labeled "100 percent pure" may contain preservatives and other chemicals, so read the label carefully and try to buy a product with the fewest ingredients possible.

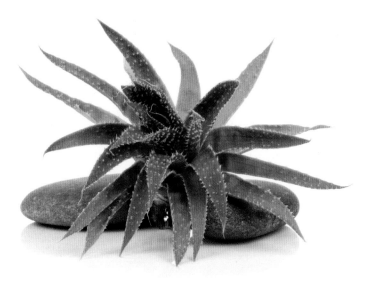

❧ SWOLLEN ANKLES ❧

Swollen ankles are fairly common, especially among older people and pregnant women. Also known as peripheral edema, it's generally caused by an accumulation of fluids and is typically painless. Due to gravity, this swelling often occurs in the lower legs and ankles. Swollen ankles can be the result of standing for long periods of time, injuring one's ankle, pregnancy or the menstrual cycle, or taking certain medications—or, it can be a symptom of a more serious underlying medical condition. If the swelling is severe or accompanied by other symptoms, see a doctor. Otherwise, try these simple home remedies to get you back into your favorite footwear once again.

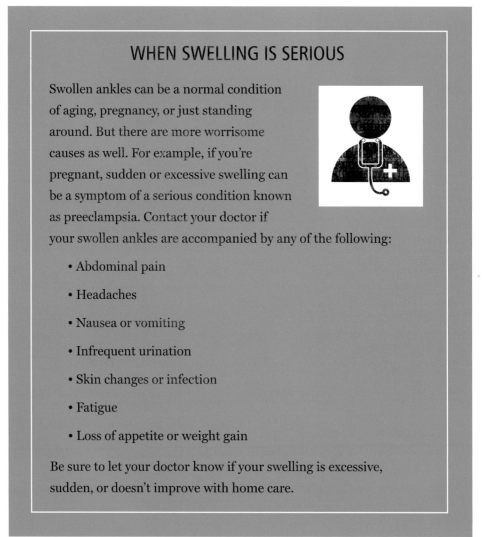

WHEN SWELLING IS SERIOUS

Swollen ankles can be a normal condition of aging, pregnancy, or just standing around. But there are more worrisome causes as well. For example, if you're pregnant, sudden or excessive swelling can be a symptom of a serious condition known as preeclampsia. Contact your doctor if your swollen ankles are accompanied by any of the following:

- Abdominal pain

- Headaches

- Nausea or vomiting

- Infrequent urination

- Skin changes or infection

- Fatigue

- Loss of appetite or weight gain

Be sure to let your doctor know if your swelling is excessive, sudden, or doesn't improve with home care.

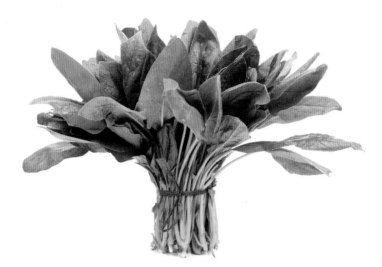

Magnesium

Edema can be a sign of a magnesium deficiency in the body. To get more of this mineral, add magnesium-rich foods—such as dark leafy greens, nuts, and beans—to your diet. Or, look for a magnesium supplement, 200 milligrams a day. However, if you're pregnant, talk to your doctor before taking a supplement.

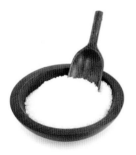

Epsom Salt

Epsom salt is made up of magnesium and sulfate. Magnesium can help eliminate fluid retention and relax muscles. Add 2 cups of Epsom salt to a tub of warm water and soak your ankles (or take a relaxing bath) for fifteen minutes.

Elevation

Since gravity is shifting fluids down to your ankles, fight this effect by elevating your legs when possible above your heart. You can use a pillow when in bed. Do this several times a day until you see results.

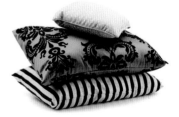

❧ TEETHING ❧

It's hard to know who has it worse—the poor baby with the angry gums, or the exhausted parent answering a cranky infant's cries in the middle of the night. According to the American Academy of Pediatrics, babies generally start teething between four and seven months of age, although this timing varies widely. Teething babies may drool, cry and fuss, have a low-grade fever, or bite or chew on whatever's handy. When your baby's going through this rite of passage, it's natural to want to ease her pain as quickly as possible. To soothe those aching gums, try the following remedies—and restore peace (and quiet) to your household once more.

Cold Washcloth

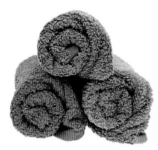

Soak a washcloth in cold water and give it to your baby to gnaw on. The cold will reduce swelling and soothe baby's gums, as will the pressure created by chewing. You can also use cold breast milk instead of water if that will make your baby more likely to try it. Or, if your child's pediatrician approves, dip the washcloth in chamomile tea, cool in the refrigerator, and give it to baby to chomp on. Chamomile is known for its soothing, pain-relieving properties.

Carrot

If your baby has started on solids, try giving him a whole carrot to gnaw on. Place a carrot in the refrigerator, and once it's cold (again, not frozen), give it to baby while you hold one end. You'll need to carefully supervise, to make sure that he doesn't choke on any little pieces that may come off. Never give your infant a baby carrot, as those are choking hazards.

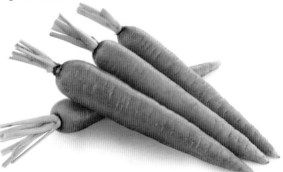

OLD WIVES TALE

An old folk remedy calls for rubbing brandy or whiskey on a teething baby's gums. While previous generations may have followed this tradition, the U.S. National Institutes of Health warns parents against this practice, which can be dangerous for baby.

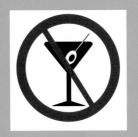

    Another traditional remedy that fails to hold up to modern standards is using ice or something frozen to soothe the pain of teething. Never give your baby anything frozen to gnaw on! Frozen teethers and other objects tend to become too hard and can damage your baby's gums.

Gum Massage

The simplest remedy for teething may be one of the most effective. Wash your hands with soap and water, and gently rub your baby's gums with your finger. The pressure from your finger can provide some much-needed relief.

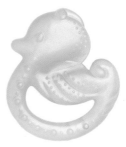

❧ TENDER BREASTS ❧

Whether they're sore, sensitive to the touch, or just plain painful, tender breasts can make exercising, sleeping, or going about your daily business uncomfortable. Breast tenderness can have various causes, including hormonal changes during the menstrual cycle or pregnancy, too much caffeine, weight gain, or medications such as birth control pills. Breast tenderness can often be relieved by wearing a more supportive bra, cutting back on caffeine, and taking over-the-counter pain relievers. And hormone-related breast pain often goes away on its own, easing up after your period, your first trimester of pregnancy, or menopause. For natural alternatives, try these home remedies to ease those tender breasts.

WARNING

If you're pregnant, be sure to consult your doctor before taking *any* medications—including overt-the-counter medicines, essential oils, and supplements. Also talk to your doctor about any potential changes to your diet.

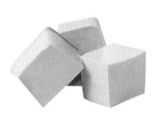

Soy

A staple in Asian countries, soy contains estrogen-like compounds called phytoestrogens that may affect hormonal shifts during menstruation and menopause—helping to relieve symptoms such as sore breasts and hot flashes. Try adding two servings of soy to your diet a day; popular options include edamame, soy milk, and tofu.

Evening Primrose Oil

A popular treatment for PMS pain, this herbal remedy may increase levels of certain fatty acids and balance the hormones, alleviating pain in the breasts. Take 3–4 grams daily by mouth.

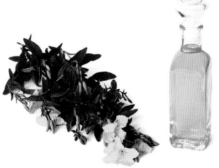

Flaxseeds

Flaxseeds are another source of phytoestrogens, which may reduce the amount of estrogen your body naturally produces, causing less breast tenderness. Grind up 2 tablespoons of flaxseeds in your blender and sprinkle on top of smoothies, salads, or other cold meals each day. Do not add flaxseeds to hot foods or beverages.

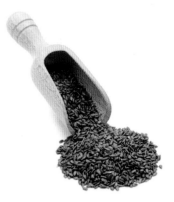

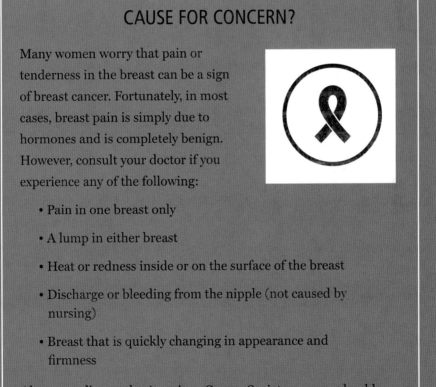

CAUSE FOR CONCERN?

Many women worry that pain or tenderness in the breast can be a sign of breast cancer. Fortunately, in most cases, breast pain is simply due to hormones and is completely benign. However, consult your doctor if you experience any of the following:

- Pain in one breast only

- A lump in either breast

- Heat or redness inside or on the surface of the breast

- Discharge or bleeding from the nipple (not caused by nursing)

- Breast that is quickly changing in appearance and firmness

Also, according to the American Cancer Society, women should begin learning about breast self-exams in their twenties, and start receiving yearly mammograms at age forty.

𝒯 TENDER GUMS 𝒴

Sore, painful, or tender gums can have many causes. Overly vigorous brushing can damage the gums. Pregnancy, menstruation, and birth control pills cause hormonal changes that can lead to tender gums and bleeding upon brushing. Other causes may include gingivitis, a mild form of gum disease caused by bacteria under the gumline; more serious gum disease, known as periodontitis; canker sores; receding gums; tobacco use; and dentures that don't fit properly. Good oral hygiene, such as proper brushing and flossing, can eliminate some causes of gum tenderness. Several home remedies can also relieve the discomfort of sore, tender gums and bring a smile to your face once more.

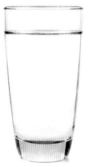

Salt Water

A warm salt water rinse can ease inflammation of the gums; in addition, salt is a natural disinfectant. Dissolve ¼–½ teaspoon of salt in an 8-ounce glass of warm water, and use the solution as a rinse, as you would mouthwash. This is a short-term solution, however; rinsing daily with salt water for longer than two to three weeks is not recommended, as the alkaline nature of the salt water can erode and soften the enamel on the teeth.

Baking Soda

Baking soda can prevent the formation of plaque, a cause of gum disease. Many toothpastes include baking soda, or you can mix baking soda with enough water to form a paste, and brush with the mixture. Rinse with water to remove any residue from the mouth.

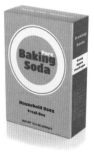

VISIT THE DENTIST

Gum tenderness often isn't anything serious. But if improving your oral hygiene doesn't ease your symptoms, a trip to the dentist may be in order. Consult your dentist if you have any of the following symptoms:

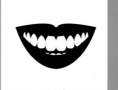

- Red, swollen gums

- Persistent bad breath

- Bleeding upon brushing

- Receding gums

Make sure to schedule an oral exam and cleaning twice a year, and always let your dentist know about any gum or tooth pain you're experiencing.

Hydrogen Peroxide

Hydrogen peroxide has anti-bacterial properties that can reduce plaque formation and help treat the gingivitis that's often behind sore, tender gums. Mix 3 percent hydrogen peroxide (found at pharmacies and the dental aisle in some drugstores) with an equal amount of water and use as a mouthwash. Do not swallow the mixture.

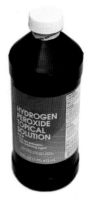

✍ TENDINITIS AND BURSITIS ✍

Tendinitis and bursitis cause inflammation or breakdown of tissue around your muscles and bones. Tendons are fibrous bands connecting muscles to bones; bursas are thin, fluid-filled sacs that reduce friction by cushioning bones from other moving body parts, such as muscles, tendons, or skin. When injury or overuse causes a tendon or bursa to swell, severe pain can follow—most often in the knees, elbows, wrists, hips, or ankles. Tendinitis and bursitis are common in certain sports (i.e., "tennis elbow") or jobs requiring repetitive motion, such as prolonged use of tools. These conditions can even be caused by kneeling on a hard surface for too long. According to the American College of Rheumatology, persistent pain may require nonsteroidal anti-inflammatory drugs (NSAIDs) such as aspirin or ibuprofen, supports, physical therapy, or even surgery. However, for mild cases of bursitis or tendinitis, often home care is enough to ease your pain and put you on the path to recovery.

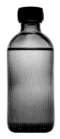

Castor Oil

Castor oil also fights inflammation, and combined with heat, provides powerful pain relief. Apply the castor oil to a cloth and place it on the affected area. Cover the entire area with plastic wrap. Apply a heating pad for an hour. Repeat this process four to five nights a week until the pain subsides.

CALL YOUR DOCTOR

Occasionally tendinitis and bursitis can become more serious. Call your doctor if you're suddenly unable to move a joint, pain continues to worsen, you see signs of infection (such as redness or swelling), or your condition persists longer than three to six weeks.

Omega-3 Fatty Acids

The omega-3 fatty acids found in certain fish, such as sardines, tuna, and mackerel, have anti-inflammatory properties. Add two servings of fish a week to your diet (plant-based sources such as tofu or walnuts are also beneficial), or add fish oil capsules to your supplement regimen.

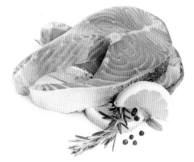

RICE

For the first twenty-four to forty-eight hours, reduce pain and inflammation with the RICE method:

- **Rest.** Rest the injured area and avoid activity that places weight on it.
- **Ice.** Wrap ice in a cloth and apply to the injury for ten to fifteen minutes at a time, once or twice a day.
- **Compression.** Use an elastic wrap to snugly wrap the area, making sure not to cut off circulation.
- **Elevation.** Keep the injured area elevated above your heart when possible.

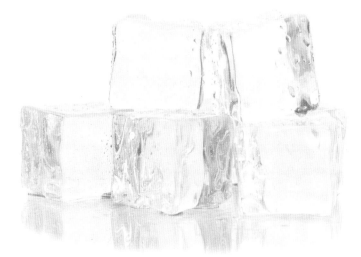

❧ TINNITUS ❧

That ringing in your ears may be tinnitus, the perception of sound in one or both ears not caused by an external source. According to the American Academy of Otolaryngology—Head and Neck Surgery, 50 million Americans have experienced tinnitus. Tinnitus is a symptom of an underlying condition, generally age-related hearing loss, although it can also be caused by excessive ear wax, middle-ear infections, medications that damage hair cells in the inner ear, and other conditions. Many cases of tinnitus improve on their own with time; however, more persistent cases may require treatment of the underlying condition, hearing aids, antidepressants, or devices that emit low-level white noise to mask symptoms. If your tinnitus interferes with your life, comes on suddenly, or is accompanied by dizziness, visit your physician (as you should if you notice any loss of hearing). You can also try these natural remedies to once again enjoy the sounds of silence.

LIFESTYLE CHANGES

Certain lifestyle changes can help to manage that noise in your head. Avoid or reduce these factors that can aggravate your tinnitus:

- Excessive or loud noise

- Caffeine

- Smoking

- Alcohol use

- Stress

In addition, you can sometimes reduce symptoms with daily exercise and by masking the sounds with white noise, such as a fan or the hum of an air conditioner.

Ginkgo Biloba

Ginkgo biloba, used in Chinese medicine, is a popular alternative treatment for tinnitus, touted for its ability to improve blood flow. However, its effectiveness is disputed, and it will likely help your tinnitus only if its underlying cause is related to circulatory problems. Ginkgo is available as a supplement, with recommended dosages up to 240 milligrams a day. Ginkgo may interfere with certain medications, so talk to your doctor before beginning a supplement.

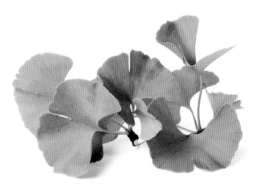

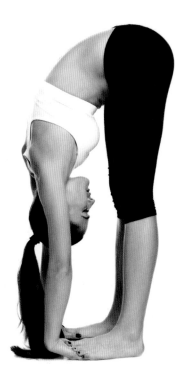

Exercise

Exercise can improve circulation and reduce stress—both of which may offer relief of tinnitus and are frequently recommend to those suffering with this condition. Since stress can aggravate tinnitus, one effective form of exercise is yoga, which is mentally relaxing in addition to a physical workout. Avoid high-impact aerobic activities that involve jumping and jarring the head, as these may actually worsen your tinnitus.

✈ TOOTH STAINS ✈

The song goes "you're never fully dressed without a smile"—but it can be hard to display your smile to the world when your teeth are discolored. Tooth stains can be caused by many factors, including tobacco use, poor dental hygiene, regular coffee drinking, or certain medications. Tooth discoloration can also accompany aging, as the enamel on the teeth gradually wears away. Brushing and flossing, as well as regular cleanings from your dentist, can help keep your teeth white by removing plaque and stain-causing foods and beverages. You can also invest in over-the-counter whitening products, or whitening procedures at the dentist's office. For simple (and cheap) alternatives, try these at-home treatments that will bring a smile to your face.

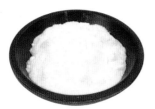

Baking Soda

An ingredient in many toothpaste brands, baking soda scrubs away plaque and surface stains to restore a healthy shine to your teeth. Mix a little baking soda with enough water to form a paste, and brush your teeth with the mixture. Rinse with water to remove any residue from the mouth.

Seeds and Nuts

These hard, naturally abrasive foods can scrape plaque and stains off of teeth. They're also full of protein and healthy for you. So enjoy some seeds and nuts as an afternoon snack—and remove some of the residue that's built up on your pearly whites throughout the day.

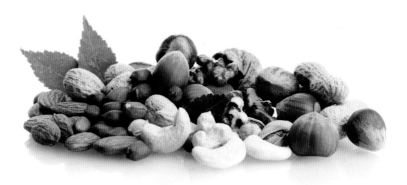

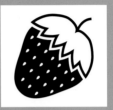

THE STRAWBERRY MYTH

One popular "whitening method" is to rub mashed-up strawberries on your teeth. The belief is that the acids in the berries dissolve stains. However, in a recent study, a researcher at the University of Iowa tested this theory by rubbing a mixture of strawberries and baking soda on twenty recently extracted human molars for five minutes at a time, three times daily for ten days—and discovered no actual whitening effect. The harsh acids did wear down the teeth's surface hardness, unfortunately, making them vulnerable to other dental problems.

Sugarless Gum

Chewing gum stimulates saliva production, which helps to remove food particles from teeth and protect teeth from stains. Sugarless gums containing xylitol also battle bacteria, which can contribute to bad breath, cavities, and other oral health problems.

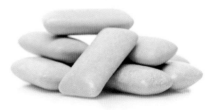

❧ TOOTHACHES ❧

When you have a toothache, it can be hard to concentrate on anything other than that nagging pain in your mouth. A toothache occurs when the part of the tooth containing nerve endings becomes irritated or inflamed. This is often the result of tooth decay and resulting cavities—which may cause you to feel pain upon eating or drinking something cold or hot. Other causes may include gum disease, infection, or an injury to a tooth. Since a toothache is often the first sign of a cavity or infection, it's a good idea to get it checked out by your dentist, who may need to fill the cavity, prescribe antibiotics, or perform other procedures. While you wait for your appointment, or to deal with pain that's not the result of a cavity or other issue, you can try these home remedies to help you chew in peace once again.

Clove Oil

Clove oil has anesthetic properties, due to the presence of eugenol, a chemical compound known to dull pain. In a 2006 study published in the *Journal of Dentistry*, clove oil was shown to numb tissue as well as benzocaine, an ingredient found in over-the-counter tooth pain relievers. Apply a small amount of clove oil to a cotton swab and apply to the affected area. Make sure to use small amounts, as large quantities of clove oil may cause liver and respiratory problems when ingested.

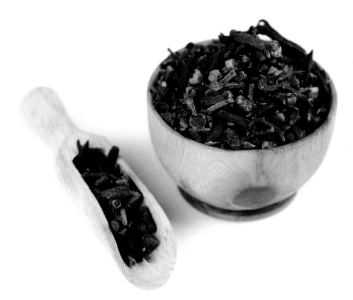

Salt Water

Rinsing with warm salt water can reduce inflammation and act against bacteria. Dissolve one ¼–½ teaspoon of salt in an 8-ounce glass of warm water, and use the solution as a rinse, as you would mouthwash. This is a short-term solution, however; rinsing daily with salt water for longer than two to three weeks is not recommended, as the alkaline nature of the salt water can erode and soften the enamel on the teeth.

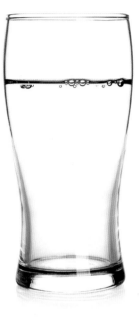

MORE THAN AN ACHE

Sometimes tooth pain indicates a more serious infection. Contact your dentist right away if your toothache is accompanied by fever, swelling of the gums or face, severe pain more than two days after an extraction, a facial rash, difficulty swallowing, headaches, dizziness, or nausea

❧ ULCERS ❧

An ulcer is a hole in the lining of the gastrointestinal tract, generally in the stomach or upper part of the small intestine. Ulcers in the stomach are called gastric ulcers, while ulcers in the small intestine are known as duodenal ulcers. Symptoms usually begin with mild pain that grows more intense if left untreated, and, less commonly, bleeding, loss of appetite, and vomiting. Ulcers used to be attributed to excessive stress or a genetic predisposition. Today, experts believe ulcers are caused by bacterial infection, or by extended use of certain pain medications, such as aspirin or ibuprofen, that wear away at the stomach lining. Doctors typically treat ulcers with antibiotics (if bacteria are present) or medications that inhibit stomach acid production. Your doctor may also recommend an over-the-counter antacid for pain relief. While you're treating your ulcer, try these simple home remedies to relieve the symptoms of this often-painful condition.

LIFESTYLE CHANGES

To help prevent or avoid aggravating an ulcer:

- **Avoid alcohol and smoking**. Both of these are harmful to the stomach lining.

- **Reduce stress.** Stress many not cause ulcers, but it can make them worse.

- **Eat fiber.** Small, frequent meals rich in fiber can help to protect the digestive lining from stomach acids.

Talk to your doctor about how diet and lifestyle changes can ease the pain of your ulcer.

Probiotics

Probiotics can repopulate the digestive tract with "good" bacteria to balance out the bad, such as the *H. pylori* bacteria often present with ulcers. Look for probiotic supplements, or add probiotic-containing foods such as kefir or yogurt (containing "live active cultures") to your diet. Also add probiotics to your diet when taking antibiotics, to maintain the balance of bacteria in your digestive system.

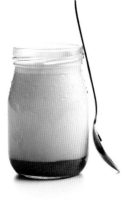

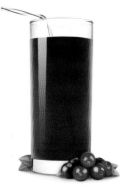

Cranberry Juice

Often used as a treatment for urinary tract infections, cranberry juice also may be effective for people suffering from ulcers. Studies have shown that compounds in cranberry juice, known as proanthocyanidins, prevent *H. pylori* from adhering to the stomach lining. Drink 1 cup of cranberry juice per day, or take a cranberry supplement (400 milligrams, twice a day).

Licorice

Licorice has been shown to kill *H. pylori* bacteria and may help protect the stomach lining against damage from nonsteroidal anti-inflammatory drugs (NSAIDs), such as aspirin or ibuprofen. Look for DGL-licorice, which has gone through a process to remove glycyrrhizin, a chemical with potentially harmful side effects. Available as a supplement, take 250 to 500 milligrams, three times daily, either an hour before or two hours after meals.

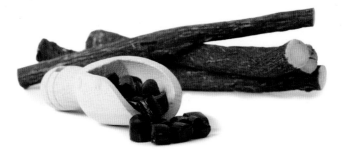

➤ URINARY TRACT INFECTIONS ➤

A urinary tract infection—commonly called a UTI—is a bacterial infection of the urinary system, the part of the body responsible for making, storing, and excreting urine. A UTI most often occurs in the bladder or urethra, although it can also affect the kidneys or ureters, tubes that transport urine from the kidneys to the bladder. Bacteria can enter the urinary tract in various ways: improper wiping after a bowel movement, holding one's urine, and sexual intercourse can all lead to infection, as can certain medical conditions. Symptoms may include painful urination, a constant urge to urinate, foul-smelling or bloody urine, or lower back pain. Because UTIs can be dangerous should they spread to your kidneys, it's important to contact your doctor if you have symptoms, as you may need antibiotics. However, there are various home remedies that can help to prevent UTIs, and that can ease your symptoms while your doctor treats the infection.

Cranberry Juice

While cranberry juice won't cure your UTI, compounds in cranberries make it difficult for bacteria—specifically *E. coli*—to connect with other bacteria and adhere to the bladder wall, reducing the risk of developing a UTI. Look for a juice that is 100 percent cranberry juice for the best effects. Drink 1 cup of cranberry juice per day, or take a cranberry supplement (400 milligrams, twice a day).

Probiotics

Probiotics can balance out "bad" bacteria with "good" bacteria, preventing harmful bacteria like *E. coli* from proliferating. Look for probiotic supplements, or add probiotic-containing foods such as kefir or yogurt (containing "live active cultures") to your diet. Also be sure to consume probiotics when taking antibiotics, to maintain the balance of bacteria in your body.

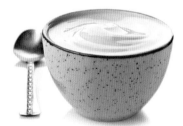

Water

Drink lots of water throughout the day to dilute your urine and flush out the infection. The less concentrated your urine is, the less it may hurt when you urinate. You can also add ¼–½ teaspoon baking soda to 1 cup of cold water, and drink it to neutralize acids in your urine, making for less painful urination.

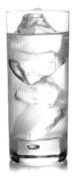

HOW TO AVOID A UTI

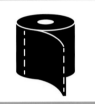

Perhaps the best way to deal with a UTI is to avoid one in the first place. While this is often easier said than done, there are certain steps you can take to protect yourself:

- Always urinate when you need to—don't hold your urine.

- Wipe from front to back, especially after a bowel movement.

- Urinate as soon as possible after sexual intercourse to flush out bacteria.

- Avoid feminine hygiene products that may upset the nature bacterial balance in the vagina, such as douches and sprays.

- Opt for panties with a cotton crotch, to avoid trapping moisture that can be a breeding ground for bacteria.

By practicing proper hygiene, staying hydrated, and urinating when you feel the urge, you can reduce your risk of developing this painful infection.

❧ VARICOSE VEINS ❧

Varicose veins—or veins which appear twisted, enlarged, and often blue or purple in color—are often a fact of life for seniors and pregnant women. Veins carry blood from the outer body back to the heart and lungs. When vein walls lose their elasticity, or when valves in the veins weaken, veins struggle to propel blood toward to the heart. Blood begins to flow backwards, pooling in the vein and causing swelling and discoloration (due to the lack of oxygen in the blood). The legs and feet are most commonly affected, due to gravity and the increased pressure from standing and walking. Varicose veins often occur with aging and obesity; in addition, during pregnancy, the greater volume of blood and growing uterus place more pressure on veins in the lower body. Varicose veins are sometimes accompanied by achiness, cramps, or itchiness. While medical procedures are available to treat varicose veins, often home care is enough to ease the symptoms and prevent future ones from occurring.

WARNING

Be sure to contact your doctor if you have tenderness or pain in a varicose vein, redness, or sudden swelling of the leg, as these signs may indicate an infection or blood clot. Also contact your doctor should you develop ulcers on the skin near a varicose vein.

Cayenne Pepper

Cayenne pepper boosts circulation, and the capsaicin present in cayenne can help relieve pain. Add a teaspoon of cayenne pepper to warm water and drink three times a day for a month.

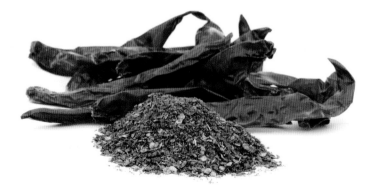

TRY THIS AT HOME

You may be able to reduce and prevent varicose veins with some simple lifestyle changes:

- Lose weight

- Exercise daily

- Don't sit or stand for long periods of time

- Wear compression stockings

These steps can take pressure off your veins and get your blood flowing—helping to avoid unsightly varicose veins.

Horse Chestnut Seed Extract

Horse chestnut seed extract is sometimes used to treat chronic venous insufficiency, a blood circulation problem that can cause varicose veins. A standard dosage is 300 milligrams of horse chestnut seed extract, containing 50 milligrams of aescin, taken two times a day.

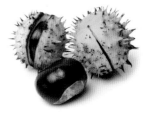

WARNING

Never eat raw horse chestnut plants or their seeds, as they can be toxic. Instead, use a standardized seed extract. Talk to your doctor if you have a bleeding disorder or are taking any medications.

⟪ WARTS ⟫

Warts are benign skin growths that occur after exposure to human papillomavirus, or HPV. While warts can occur anywhere on the body, they typically appear on the hands, feet, face, or genitals, depending on the type of wart. Warts are contagious, and can be passed to others by direct contact, sex, or by handling a contaminated towel or other object. While some warts are painless, others can itch and cause discomfort. While warts sometimes go away on their own, others can take months or years to disappear, and some never go away at all. Doctors frequently remove warts with chemical treatments or cryotherapy (freezing). If you want to avoid these procedures, salicylic acid is available in various over-the-counter products—or, you can try some readily available home remedies to get rid of that embarrassing wart.

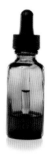

Tea Tree Oil

Tea tree oil has natural antiviral, antibacterial, and antifungal properties. Place 1 drop of undiluted tea tree oil on the wart and cover with a bandage. Leave on overnight. Remove the bandage and clean the area in the morning. Repeat this process nightly over the course of a few weeks, until the wart falls off or goes away.

WHEN TO CALL THE DOCTOR

Never try any home remedies or over-the-counter treatments on warts on the face or genitals without first talking to a doctor. If a wart persists for months and your at-home treatment isn't working, you should consider seeing a doctor. Though most warts will go away on their own, it could take years for that to happen, and in that time, you may spread the wart to other parts of your body or other people.

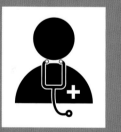

Apple Cider Vinegar

Highly acidic apple cider vinegar wears down warts; when ACV is applied to the wart, it should eventually turn black and peel off the skin. Soak a cotton ball in ACV and apply it directly to the wart. Secure it in place with a bandage or gauze. Remove the bandage and cotton ball in the morning. Repeat this process every night for a week or until you see results. If the ACV is too harsh, you can try diluting it with a little water.

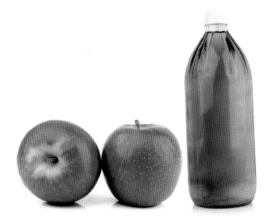

Banana Peel

Banana peels contain compounds that erode warts. Cut up a banana peel and place a piece directly on the wart, with the "mushy" side down against the wart. Secure it in place with tape. Leave on overnight and wash off the area in the morning. Repeat each night until you see results.

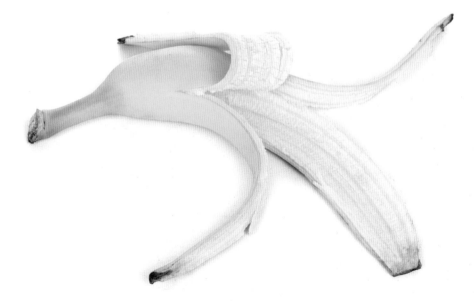

❧ WRINKLES ❧

Just because you accept that you're aging, doesn't mean you want to advertise it to the world. Wrinkles are lines or folds that appear on the skin, such as on the face around the eyes or mouth. As you age, the inner layer of skin becomes thinner, making skin less elastic; in addition, aging skin tends to be drier and heal more slowly. Other factors, such as exposure to the sun and smoking, can also contribute to developing wrinkles. Certain over-the-counter and prescription creams are available to smooth out wrinkles, and your dermatologist can recommend other procedures as well, such as laser treatments and chemical peels. If you want to avoid the expense and side effects that may accompany these treatments, try these natural alternatives instead.

Coconut Oil

This home remedy counteracts many of the causes of wrinkles—and smells great, too! Coconut oil is rich in antioxidants that help to protect against free radicals that can damage the skin. It's also a great moisturizer and has antifungal and antibacterial properties that can protect skin against infection. To take advantage of this oil, rub a tablespoon onto the wrinkled area of skin twice a day.

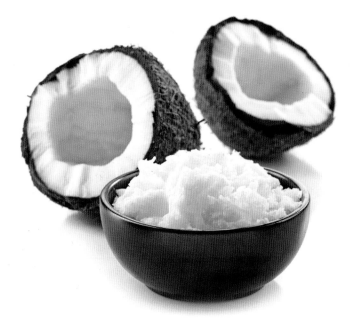

SHEDDING LIGHT ON WRINKLES

Few things prematurely age your skin like exposure to ultraviolet (UV) rays. UV light damages your skin's connective tissue, which makes skin weaker and less flexible. Limit your exposure to the sun during its peak times (between 10 a.m. and 4 p.m.), always wear a broad-spectrum sunscreen with an SPF of 30 or higher, and cover exposed skin with clothing when you can.

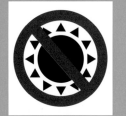

Olive Oil

Olive oil moisturizes dry skin, and its antioxidants help protect the skin from the damaging effects of the sun. Olive oil also contains a fatty acid called oleic acid, which helps the cells absorb essential fatty acids more efficiently, which can help prevent loose, saggy skin. Massage the olive oil onto the affected skin twice a day.

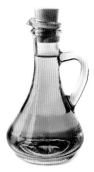

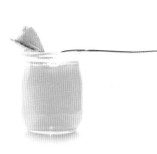

Yogurt

Plain yogurt is rich in minerals and vitamins such as ribo-flavin, which protects the skin from free-radical damage and promotes healthy cell growth. It also contains lactic acid, which exfoliates and moisturizes the skin. Spread 1–2 teaspoons of plain, unsweetened yogurt on your face as a mask. Leave on for fifteen minutes, and then rinse. You can add some mashed-up banana to the mask for extra antioxidant power.

❧ YEAST INFECTIONS ❧

While no one likes to discuss vaginal yeast infections, they are fairly common. In fact, according to the Office on Women's Health at the U.S. Department of Health and Human Services, around 75 percent of women have had a yeast infection. Also known as vaginal candidiasis, a yeast infection is an irritation of the vagina and surrounding vulva caused by an overgrowth of the fungus *Candida albicans*. Symptoms typically include itching, burning, swelling, and a thick, white vaginal discharge resembling cottage cheese. Yeast infections have various triggers, ranging from sugary foods to hormonal changes to use of certain medications such as antibiotics. While over-the-counter and prescription antifungal creams and tablets are available to treat yeast infections, you can also relieve uncomfortable symptoms with some natural alternatives.

TALK TO YOUR DOCTOR

While drugstore shelves are lined with products to cure your yeast infection, you should talk to your doctor if you've never previously been diagnosed with a yeast infection, you're pregnant, or you have recurring yeast infections. According to studies, ⅔ of women who purchase these products don't actually have a yeast infection. Treating yourself incorrectly may cause you to miss a more worrisome problem.

Probiotics

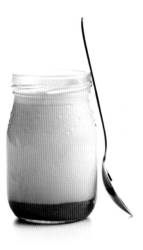

There is a delicate balance of microorganisms in the vagina. The bacteria *Lactobacillus* suppresses the growth of candida; when this balance is disrupted, an overgrowth can occur, leading to infection. Probiotics containing *Lactobacillus*—especially *Lactobacillus acidophilus*—and other "good" bacteria may help to restore this balance and prevent yeast infections. Look for probiotic supplements, or add probiotic-containing foods such as kefir or yogurt (containing "live active cultures") to your diet. Many women add probiotics to their diets when taking antibiotics, to maintain the balance of bacteria in the body.

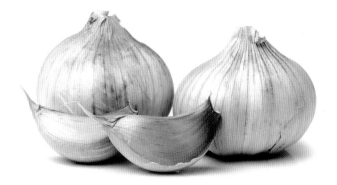

Garlic

With its natural antifungal properties, garlic is another popular treatment with primarily anecdotal evidence to support it. To give it a try, peel a fresh clove and insert it into your vagina before going to bed. Remove and flush the clove in the morning. For easier retrieval, you can sew a string through the center of the clove before inserting.

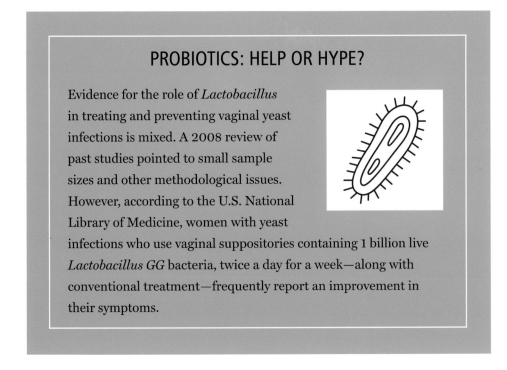

PROBIOTICS: HELP OR HYPE?

Evidence for the role of *Lactobacillus* in treating and preventing vaginal yeast infections is mixed. A 2008 review of past studies pointed to small sample sizes and other methodological issues. However, according to the U.S. National Library of Medicine, women with yeast infections who use vaginal suppositories containing 1 billion live *Lactobacillus GG* bacteria, twice a day for a week—along with conventional treatment—frequently report an improvement in their symptoms.

BIBLIOGRAPHY

Alleyne, Richard. "Secret to a Good Hangover: Honey on Toast." The *Telegraph* online, December 23, 2010. http://www.telegraph.co.uk/news/health/8222490/Secret-to-a-smooth-hangover-honey-on-toast.html.

American Academy of Dermatology. "Could Probiotics Be the Next Big Thing in Acne and Rosacea Treatments?" February 3, 2014. https://www.aad.org/stories-and-news/news-releases/could-probiotics-be-the-next-big-thing-in-acne-and-rosacea-treatments.

———. "Poison Ivy: Tips for Treating and Preventing." Accessed March 26, 2015. https://www.aad.org/dermatology-a-to-z/diseases-and-treatments/m---p/poison-ivy/tips.

American Academy of Orthopaedic Surgeons. "Sprains and Strains: What's the Difference?" Last reviewed October 2007. http://orthoinfo.aaos.org/topic.cfm?topic=A00111.

American Academy of Otolaryngology—Head and Neck Surgery. "Snoring and Sleep Apnea." Accessed March 26, 2015. http://www.entnet.org/content/snoring-and-sleep-apnea.

American Academy of Podiatric Management. "Smelly Feet and Foot Odor." Accessed March 23, 2015. http://www.aappm.org/library/1932/SmellyFeetandFootOdor.html.

American Cancer Society. "American Cancer Society Guidelines for the Early Detection of Cancer." Last revised October 29, 2014. http://www.cancer.org/healthy/findcancerearly/cancerscreeningguidelines/american-cancer-society-guidelines-for-the-early-detection-of-cancer.

American Chemical Society. "Chamomile Tea: New Evidence Supports Health Benefits." ScienceDaily, accessed February 23, 2015. www.sciencedaily.com/releases/2005/01/050104112140.htm.

American College of Rheumatology. "Tendinitis and Bursitis." Updated February 2013. https://www.rheumatology.org/Practice/Clinical/Patients/Diseases_And_Conditions/Tendinitis_and_Bursitis/.

American Heart Association. "High blood pressure causing more deaths despite drop in heart disease, stroke deaths." December 19, 2014. http://blog.heart.org/high-blood-pressure-causing-deaths-despite-drop-heart-disease-stroke-deaths/.

American Pregnancy Association. "Hyperemesis Gravidarum." Last updated June 2014. http://americanpregnancy.org/pregnancy-complications/hyperemesis-gravidarum/.

Ash Center for Comprehensive Medicine. "Cold Sores." Accessed March 22, 2015. http://ashcenter.com/conditions/cold-sores/.

Barrons, R. and D. Tassone. "Use of Lactobacillus Probiotics for Bacterial Genitourinary Infections in Women: A Review." *Clinical Therapeutics* 30, no. 3 (March 2008): 453–68. doi: 10.1016/j.clinthera.2008.03.013.

Beck, Leslie. "What Foods Should I Eat to Manage My Hot Flashes?" The *Globe and Mail* online, updated March 25, 2014. http://www.theglobeandmail.com/life/health-and-fitness/ask-a-health-expert/what-foods-should-i-eat-to-help-manage-my-hot-flashes/article17619393/.

Brown, Stephanie. "How to Make Your Own Oatmeal Bath." About.com Parenting, accessed March 22, 2015. http://babyparenting.about.com/cs/healthissues/a/oatmealbath.htm.

Calderone, Julia. "Fact or Fiction?: A Clove of Garlic Can Stop a Vaginal Yeast Infection." *Scientific American* online, October 3, 2014. http://www.scientificamerican.com/article/fact-or-fiction-a-clove-of-garlic-can-stop-a-vaginal-yeast-infection/.

Carson, C. F. et al. "Melaleuca alternifolia (Tea Tree) Oil: A Review of Antimicrobial and Other Medicinal Properties." *Clinical Microbiology Reviews* 19, no. 1 (January 2006): 50–62. doi: 10.1128/CMR.19.1.50-62.2006.

Case-Lo, Christine. "The Link Between Zinc and Erectile Dysfunction." Healthline.com, March 19, 2014. http://www.healthline.com/health/erectile-dysfunction/zinc#WhatIsZinc?1.

Centers for Disease Control and Prevention. "Infectious Diseases at School." Last reviewed and updated November 17, 2011. http://www.cdc.gov/healthyyouth/infectious/.

———. "Monitoring the Impact of Varicella Vaccination." Last reviewed and updated August 30, 2012. http://www.cdc.gov/chickenpox/hcp/monitoring-varicella.html.

Chithra P., G. B. Sajithlal, and G. Chandrakasan. "Influence of Aloe Vera on Collagen Characteristics in Healing Dermal Wounds in Rats." *Molecular and Cellular Biochemistry* 18, no. 1–2 (April 1998): 71–76. http://www.ncbi.nlm.nih.gov/pubmed/9562243.

Choi, Charles Q. "Do DIY Teeth Whitening Methods Really Work?." LiveScience.com, October 27, 2014. http://www.livescience.com/48472-teeth-whitening-methods-really-work.html.

DeNoon, Daniel J. "Coffee-Swilling Men Get Less Gout, Study Shows." WebMD.com, May 25, 2007. http://www.webmd.com/arthritis/news/20070525/coffee-lowers-gout-risk.

Dillner, Luisa. "How Safe Are Contact Lenses?" The *Guardian* online, November 23, 2014. http://www.theguardian.com/lifeandstyle/2014/nov/23/how-safe-are-contact-lenses.

DoctorOz.com. "All-Natural Headache Cures." January 9, 2012. http://www.doctoroz.com/article/all-natural-headache-cures.

———. "Bloating 101: How to Beat a Bulging Belly." August 15, 2011. http://www.doctoroz.com/article/bloating-101-how-beat-bulging-belly?page=3.

———. "Daily Dose: Magnesium." September 21, 2012. http://www.doctoroz.com/article/daily-dose-magnesium.

———. "Daily Dose: Zinc." October 14, 2009. http://www.doctoroz.com/article/daily-dose-zinc.

———. "Kitchen Cures Your Doctor Can't Live Without." April 9, 2012. http://www.doctoroz.com/article/kitchen-cures-your-doctor-can-not-live-without.

Doheny, Kathleen. "Soy Supplements Can Cool Hot Flashes: Study." WebMD.com, April 9, 2012. http://www.webmd.com/menopause/news/20120409/soy-supplements-can-cool-hot-flashes-study?page=1.

DrWeil.com. "Diarrhea," March 22, 2015. http://www.drweil.com/drw/u/ART00344/diarrhea.html.

———. "Gout." Accessed March 23, 2015. http://www.drweil.com/drw/u/ART00368/Gout.html.

———. "Is Peppermint Safe During Pregnancy?" Reviewed March 9, 2010. http://www.drweil.com/drw/u/QAA366713/Is-Peppermint-Safe-During-Pregnancy.html.

Editors of Consumer Guide. "15 Home Remedies for Calluses and Corns." HowStuffWorks.com, January 15, 2007. http://health.howstuffworks.com/wellness/natural-medicine/home-remedies/home-remedies-for-calluses-and-corns.htm.

Editors of Prevention. *The Doctor's Book of Home Remedies.* New York: Rodale, 2009.

Ellis, Mary Ellen. "Sinus Stricken? Symptoms of an Infection." Healthline.com, September 13, 2013. http://www.healthline.com/health/cold-flu/sinus-infection-symptoms#Overview1.

Evangelista, M. T. P., Abad-Casintahan, F. and Lopez-Villafuerte, L. "The effect of topical virgin coconut oil on SCORAD index, transepidermal water loss, and skin capacitance in mild to moderate pediatric atopic dermatitis: a randomized, double-blind, clinical trial." *International Journal of Dermatology* 53 (2014): 100–108. doi: 10.1111/ijd.12339.

Evans, Lindsay. "Home Remedies for Chafed Skin." AZCentral.com, accessed March 22, 2015. http://healthyliving.azcentral.com/home-remedies-chafed-skin-1853.html.

FamilyDoctor.org. "BRAT Diet: Recovering from an Upset Stomach," reviewed and updated February 2011. http://familydoctor.org/familydoctor/en/prevention-wellness/food-nutrition/weight-loss/brat-diet-recovering-from-an-upset-stomach.html.

Galland, Leo, MD. "Cherries for Health: Better Than Aspirin?" The Huffington Post, June 11, 2011. http://www.huffingtonpost.com/leo-galland-md/cherry-season-fight-pain-_b_844654.html.

Gever, John. "Vitamin D Eases Menstrual Cramps." MedPage Today, February 27, 2012. http://www.medpagetoday.com/OBGYN/GeneralOBGYN/31388.

Goodall, Claire. "11 Remedies to Get Rid of Canker Sores." EverydayRoots.com, accessed March 22, 2015. http://everydayroots.com/canker-sore-remedies.

Griffin, R. Morgan. "How Fiber Protects Your Heart." WebMD.com, October 29, 2010. http://www.webmd.com/diet/fiber-health-benefits-11/fiber-heart.

Harding, Anne. "Erectile Dysfunction? Try Losing Weight." CNN.com, August 5, 2011. http://www.cnn.com/2011/HEALTH/08/05/erectile.dysfunction.lose.weight/.

HealthyChildren.org (from the American Academy of Pediatrics). "Signs and Symptoms of Fever." Last updated June 27, 2014. http://www.healthychildren.org/English/health-issues/conditions/fever/Pages/Signs-and-Symptoms-of-Fever.aspx.

———. "Sore Throat." Last revised August 1, 2011. http://www.healthychildren.org/English/tips-tools/Symptom-Checker/Pages/Sore-Throat.aspx.

———. "Teething: 4 to 7 Months." Last updated February 23, 2015. http://www.healthychildren.org/English/ages-stages/baby/teething-tooth-care/Pages/Teething-4-to-7-Months.aspx.

———. "When to Call the Pediatrician: Fever." Last updated November 4, 2014. http://www.healthychildren.org/English/health-issues/conditions/fever/Pages/When-to-Call-the-Pediatrician.aspx.

Heller, Daniel, ND. "Magnesium: Why You Need It." DoctorOz.com, July 30, 2012. http://www.doctoroz.com/blog/daniel-heller-nd/magnesium-miracle-mineral.

Hong, Bumsik et al. "A Double-Blind Crossover Study Evaluating the Efficacy of Korean Red Ginseng in Patients With Erectile Dysfunction: A Preliminary Report." *The Journal of Urology* 168, no. 5 (November 2002): 2070–73. DOI: http://dx.doi.org/10.1016/S0022-5347(05)64298-X.

Hope, Jenny. "Garlic can lower blood pressure by 10%... but only if you take it in tablet form." The *Daily Mail* online, September 13, 2013. http://www.dailymail.co.uk/news/article-2420421/Garlic-lower-blood-pressure-10---tablet-form.html.

International Foundation for Functional Gastrointestinal Disorders. "Irritable Bowel Syndrome Statistics." Last modified January 17, 2013. http://www.aboutibs.org/site/what-is-ibs/facts/statistics.

Jang, Dai-Ja, et al. "Red Ginseng for Treating Erectile Dysfunction: A Systematic Review." *British Journal of Clinical Pharmacology* 66, no. 4 (October 2008): 444-450. doi: 10.1111/j.1365-2125.2008.03236.x.

Jeffrey, S. L. and H. J. Belcher. "Use of Arnica to Relieve Pain After Carpal-Tunnel Release Surgery." *Alternative Therapies in Health and Medicine* 2 (March–April 2002): 66–68. http://www.ncbi.nlm.nih.gov/pubmed/11892685.

Kabat, Geoffrey. "*Natural* Does Not Mean *Safe*." Slate.com, November 26, 2012. http://www.slate.com/articles/health_and_science/medical_examiner/2012/11/herbal_supplement_dangers_fda_does_not_regulate_supplements_and_they_can.html.

Keenan, J. M. , et al. "Oat ingestion reduces systolic and diastolic blood pressure in patients with mild or borderline hypertension: a pilot trial." *The Journal of Family Practice* 51, no. 4 (April 2002): 369. http://www.ncbi.nlm.nih.gov/pubmed/11978262.

Kitchens, Simone. "Do Cucumbers Really Help With Puffy Eyes? Pros Weigh In On This Beauty Legend." The Huffington Post, October 16, 2012. http://www.huffingtonpost.com/2012/10/16/puffy-eyes-undereyes-cucumbers-cures-remedies_n_1964329.html.

Landau, Elizabeth. "From a Tree, a 'Miracle' Called Aspirin." CNN.com, December 22, 2010. http://www.cnn.com/2010/HEALTH/12/22/aspirin.history/.

Live Science Staff. "Why Does Coffee Cause Bad Breath?" LiveScience.com, April 5, 2012. http://www.livescience.com/33818-coffee-bad-breath-llmmp.html.

Mabey, Richard and Michael McIntyre. *The New Age Herbalist: How to Use Herbs for Healing, Nutrition, Body Care, and Relaxation.* New York, Simon & Schuster, 1988: 71–72.

Mayo Clinic. "Burns: First Aid." Last modified January 29, 2015. http://www.mayoclinic.org/first-aid/first-aid-burns/basics/art-20056649.

———. "Ginkgo (Ginkgo biloba): Dosing." Last updated November 1, 2013. http://www.mayoclinic.org/drugs-supplements/ginkgo/dosing/hrb-20059541.

———. "Sodium Bicarbonate: Proper Use." Last updated December 1, 2014. http://www.mayoclinic.org/drugs-supplements/sodium-bicarbonate-oral-route-intravenous-route-subcutaneous-route/proper-use/drg-20065950.

———. "Will Taking Zinc for Colds Make My Colds Go Away Faster?" March 4, 2015. http://www.mayoclinic.org/diseases-conditions/common-cold/expert-answers/zinc-for-colds/faq-20057769.

Mayo Clinic Physicians. *Mayo Clinic Book of Alternative Medicine and Home Remedies.* Oxmoor House, 2013.

McLeod, Jaime. "Natural Itch Relief." *Farmers' Almanac* online, June 6, 2011. http://farmersalmanac.com/health/2011/06/06/natural-itch-relief/.

McMullen, Laura. "Scars: Make Them Go (Mostly) Away." *US News and World Report* online, April 25, 2014. http://health.usnews.com/health-news/health-wellness/articles/2014/04/25/scars-make-them-go-mostly-away.

MedicalNewsToday.com. "Cranberries for Urinary Tract Infections—New Evidence." Last updated July 17, 2013. http://www.medicalnewstoday.com/articles/263426.php.

———. "What Are Skin Tags? What Causes Skin Tags?" Last updated February 11, 2015. http://www.medicalnewstoday.com/articles/67317.php.

MedicineNet.com. "Taking Calcium Supplements? Want To Avoid Kidney Stones?" Last reviewed July 7, 2004. http://www.medicinenet.com/script/main/art.asp?articlekey=1887&page=2.

MedlinePlus: A Service of the U.S. National Library of Medicine. "Calendula." Last modified November 13, 2014. http://www.nlm.nih.gov/medlineplus/druginfo/natural/235.html.

———. "Evening Primrose Oil." Last reviewed August 21, 2014. http://www.nlm.nih.gov/medlineplus/druginfo/natural/1006.html.

———. "Ginger." Last reviewed June 30, 2013. http://www.nlm.nih.gov/medlineplus/druginfo/natural/961.html#Action.

———. "Horse Chestnut." Last reviewed October 31, 2014. http://www.nlm.nih.gov/medlineplus/druginfo/natural/1055.html.

———. "Morning Sickness." Updated August 23, 2012. http://www.nlm.nih.gov/medlineplus/ency/patientinstructions/000604.htm.

———. "Sleep Apnea." Accessed March 26, 2015. http://www.nlm.nih.gov/medlineplus/sleepapnea.html.

———. "Valerian." Last reviewed May 30, 2014. http://www.nlm.nih.gov/medlineplus/druginfo/natural/870.html#Dosage.

Miller, K. C. et al. "Reflex Inhibition of Electrically Induced Muscle Cramps in Hypohydrated Humans." *Medicine and Science in Sports and Exercise* 42, no. 5 (May 2010): 953–61. doi: 10.1249/MSS.0b013e3181c0647e.

Moazzez, R., D. Bartlett, and A. Anggiansah. "The Effect of Chewing Sugar-Free Gum on Gastro-Esophageal Reflux." *Journal of Dental Research* 84, no. 11 (November 2005): 1062–65. http://www.ncbi.nlm.nih.gov/pubmed/16246942.

National Center for Complementary and Integrative Health. "Herbs at a Glance." Last modified March 24, 2015. https://nccih.nih.gov/health/herbsataglance.htm.

———. "Key Findings from the 2012 National Health Interview Survey." Last modified March 13, 2015. https://nccih.nih.gov/research/statistics/NHIS/2012/key-findings.

———. "Tea Tree Oil." Updated April 2012. https://nccih.nih.gov/health/tea/treeoil.htm.

National Geographic. *Complete Guide to Natural Home Remedies*. New York: National Geographic Society, 2012.

National Health Service. "Flatulence." Last reviewed April 25, 2013. http://www.nhs.uk/Conditions/Flatulence/Pages/Introduction.aspx.

National Institute of Arthritis and Musculoskeletal and Skin Diseases. "Questions and Answers About Gout." April 2012. http://www.niams.nih.gov/health_info/gout/#do.

National Institutes of Health: Office of Dietary Supplements. "Vitamin D." Last reviewed November 10, 2014. http://ods.od.nih.gov/factsheets/VitaminD-HealthProfessional/#h4.

———. "Valerian," Last reviewed March 15, 2013. http://ods.od.nih.gov/factsheets/Valerian-HealthProfessional/.

National Kidney Foundation. "Herbal and Natural Remedies." Accessed March 26, 2015. https://www.psoriasis.org/treating-psoriasis/complementary-and-alternative/herbal-remedies.

———. "Kidney Stones." Accessed March 26, 2015. https://www.kidney.org/atoz/content/kidneystones.

National Psoriasis Foundation. "Comorbities Associated with Psoriatic Disease." Accessed March 26, 2015. https://www.psoriasis.org/about-psoriasis/related-conditions.

National Rosacea Society. "Rosacea Triggers Survey." Accessed March 26, 2015. http://www.rosacea.org/patients/materials/triggersgraph.php.

New York Botanical Garden. "Healing Plants." March 26, 2015. http://www.nybg.org/wildmedicine/plants.html.

O'Connor, Anahad. "Really? The Claim: Cranberry Juice Can Cure Ulcers." The *New York Times* online, June 6, 2011. http://www.nytimes.com/2011/06/07/health/07really.html.

———. "Really? The Claim: Gargling with Salt Water Can Ease Cold Symptoms." The *New York Times* online, September 27, 2010. http://www.nytimes.com/2010/09/28/health/28real.html.

———. "Really? The Claim: A Tennis Ball on the Back of Pajamas Can Cut Snoring." The *New York Times* online, July 11, 2011. http://well.blogs.nytimes.com/2011/07/11/really-the-claim-a-tennis-ball-on-the-back-of-pajamas-can-cut-snoring/.

———. "Really? Ginseng Can Help Relieve Fatigue." The *New York Times* online, June 18, 2012. http://well.blogs.nytimes.com//2012/06/18/really-ginseng-can-help-relieve-fatigue/.

———. "Remedies: Clove Oil for Tooth Pain." The *New York Times* online, February 17, 2011. http://well.blogs.nytimes.com/2011/02/17/remedies-clove-oil-for-tooth-pain/.

Ozgoli, G., M. Goli, and M. Simbar. "Effects of Ginger Capsules on Pregnancy, Nausea, and Vomiting." *Journal of Alternative and Complementary Medicine* 15, no. 3 (March 2009): 243–46. doi: 10.1089/acm.2008.0406.

Parks, Chanel. "Razor Burn Is the Worst, So Here's How to Prevent It." The Huffington Post, January 29, 2014. http://www.huffingtonpost.com/2014/01/29/prevent-razor-burn_n_4661255.html.

Pikul, Corrie. "The Truth About All-Natural Teeth Whiteners." The Huffington Post, December 10, 2014. http://www.huffingtonpost.com/2014/12/10/natural-teeth-whiteners_n_6271062.html.

Praderio, Caroline. "Honey Heals Canker Sores?" Prevention.com, August 18, 2014. http://www.prevention.com/mind-body/natural-remedies/honey-natural-remedy-canker-sores.

Prasad, A. S. et al. "Zinc Status and Serum Testosterone Levels of Healthy Adults." *Nutrition* 12, no. 5 (May 1996): 344–48. http://www.ncbi.nlm.nih.gov/pubmed/8875519.

Rahnama, Marjan et al. "The Healing Effect of Licorice (Glycyrrhiza glabra) on Helicobacter Pylori Infected Peptic Ulcers." *The Journal of Research in Medical Sciences* 18, no. 6 (June 2013): 532–33.

Raloff, Janet. "Cinnamon Cleans the Breath." *Science News*. May 20, 2004. Cinnamon: ScienceNews.org https://www.sciencenews.org/blog/food-thought/cinnamon-cleans-breath.

Reader's Digest. *1,801 Home Remedies: Trustworthy Treatments for Everyday Health Problems.* Pleasantville, NY: The Reader's Digest Association, 2004.

Redbook.com. "12 Foods That Naturally Whiten Your Teeth." Accessed March 2666, 2015. http://www.redbookmag.com/body/advice/g667/teeth-whitening-foods/.

Rensselaer Polytechnic Institute. "Light From Self-Luminous Tablet Computers Can Affect Evening Melatonin, Delaying Sleep." August 27, 2012. http://news.rpi.edu/luwakkey/3074#sthash.Tvft66J6.dpuf.

Repinski, Karyn. "The Best Scar Treatments." *Fitness* Magazine online, accessed March 26, 2015. http://www.fitnessmagazine.com/beauty/skin-care/best-scar-treatments/.

Reynolds, Gretchen. "Can Pickle Juice Stop Muscle Cramps?" *The New York Times* online, June 9, 2010. http://well.blogs.nytimes.com/2010/06/09/phys-ed-can-pickle-juice-stop-muscle-cramps/.

Royal Society of Chemistry. "Toast with Honey Is the Little-Known But Ideal Way to Combat a Hangover." December 23, 2010. http://www.rsc.org/AboutUs/News/PressReleases/2010/Hangover.asp.

Runner's World online. "Shin Splints." Accessed March 26, 2015. http://www.runnersworld.com/tag/shin-splints.

Schofield, Kirsten. "3 Wrist Exercises to Prevent Carpal Tunnel." Healthline.com, September 3, 2014. http://www.healthline.com/health/carpal-tunnel-wrist-exercises#2.

Sears, Dr. "Ask Dr. Sears: Natural Earache Relievers." Parenting.com. Accessed March 22, 2015. http://www.parenting.com/article/ask-dr-sears-natural-earache-relievers.

Serafini, Mauro, Daniele Del Rio, Denis N'Dri Yao et al. "Health Benefits of Tea." Chapter 12 in *Herbal Medicine: Biomolecular and Clinical Aspects.* 2nd ed. Edited by I. F. F. Benzie and S. Wachtel-Galor. Boca Raton, FL: CRC Press, 2011. Available from: http://www.ncbi.nlm.nih.gov/books/NBK92768/.

Shea, Taylor. "11 Surprising Home Remedies for Burns." Reader's Digest, accessed March 22, 2015. http://www.rd.com/slideshows/home-remedies-for-burns/view-all/.

Skerrett, Patrick J. "Stopping Nosebleeds: A Pinch Will Usually Do the Trick." Harvard Health Publications, October 18, 2013. http://www.health.harvard.edu/blog/stopping-nosebleeds-a-pinch-will-usually-do-the-trick-201310186769.

Skin Cancer Foundation. "Worst-Case Scenario: Treating Sunburn." Accessed March 26, 2015. http://www.skincancer.org/prevention/sunburn/worst-case-scenario-treating-sunburn.

Stevens, Richard G. et al. "Adverse Health Effects of Nighttime Lighting." *American Journal of Preventative Medicine* 45, no. 3 (2013): 343–46. http://www.ncbi.nlm.nih.gov/pubmed/23953362

University of Maryland Medical Center. "Bursitis." Last updated May 7, 2013. http://umm.edu/health/medical/altmed/condition/bursitis.

———. "Carpal Tunnel Syndrome." Last updated May 31, 2013. http://umm.edu/health/medical/altmed/condition/carpal-tunnel-syndrome.

———. "Food Poisoning." Last updated May 7, 2013. http://umm.edu/health/medical/altmed/condition/food-poisoning.

———. "Peppermint." Last updated May 7, 2013. http://umm.edu/health/medical/altmed/herb/peppermint.

———. "Peptic Ulcer." Last updated September 3, 2013. http://umm.edu/health/medical/altmed/condition/peptic-ulcer.

———. "Warts." Last reviewed June 9, 2012. http://umm.edu/health/medical/altmed/condition/warts.

———. "Willow Bark." Last updated May 7, 2013. http://umm.edu/health/medical/altmed/herb/willow-bark.

University of Michigan Health System. "Urinary Incontinence (Holistic)." Last reviewed April 15, 2014. http://www.uofmhealth.org/health-library/hn-10007459.

U.S. Department of Health and Human Services and the U.S. Department of Agriculture. "Dietary Guidelines for Americans: Chapter 7, Carbohydrates." Updated July 9, 2008. http://www.health.gov/dietaryguidelines/dga2005/document/html/chapter7.htm.

The *Wall Street Journal* online. "The Surprising Nosebleed Fix," updated November 11, 2013. http://www.wsj.com/articles/SB10001424052702303914304579191842804420788.

Wang, Li, PhD, et al. "Effect of a Moderate Fat Diet With and Without Avocados on Lipoprotein Particle Number, Size and Subclasses in Overweight and Obese Adults: A Randomized, Controlled Trial." *JAHA: Journal of the American Heart Association* 4 (2015). doi: 10.1161/JAHA.114.001355.

Warner, Jennifer. "Low Vitamin D Levels Tied to Incontinence." WebMD.com, March 22, 2010. http://www.webmd.com/urinary-incontinence-oab/news/20100322/low-vitamin-d-linked-incontinence.

WebMD.com. "Black Cohosh for Menopause." Last updated March 12, 2014. http://www.webmd.com/menopause/guide/black-cohosh-for-menopause-symptoms-topic-overview.

———. "Cranberries and Your Health." Reviewed November 2, 2014. http://www.webmd.com/vitamins-and-supplements/lifestyle-guide-11/supplement-guide-cranberry.

———. "Dietary Fiber for Constipation." Reviewed September 4, 2014. http://www.webmd.com/digestive-disorders/dietary-fiber-the-natural-solution-for-constipation?.

———. "Manuka Honey." Reviewed February 12, 2015. http://www.webmd.com/a-to-z-guides/manuka-honey-medicinal-uses?.

———. "Sodium Bicarbonate (Baking Soda) for Kidney Stones." Last updated May 2, 3013. http://www.webmd.com/kidney-stones/sodium-bicarbonate-baking-soda-for-kidney-stones.

Whorton, James C. *Nature Cures: The History of Alternative Medicine in America*. New York: Oxford University Press, 2002.

WomensHealth.gov (US Department of Health and Human Services). "Vaginal Yeast Infections Fact Sheet." Last updated December 23, 2014. http://www.womenshealth.gov/publications/our-publications/fact-sheet/vaginal-yeast-infections.html.

World Health Organization. "Healthy Diet." Updated January 2015. http://www.who.int/mediacentre/factsheets/fs394/en/.

———. "WHO Traditional Medicine Strategy: 2014-2023." Accessed March 26, 2015. http://apps.who.int/iris/bitstream/10665/92455/1/9789241506090_eng.pdf.

Woznicki, Katrina. "Cranberry Juice Fights Urinary Tract Infections Quickly." WebMD.com, August 23, 2010. http://www.webmd.com/women/news/20100823/cranberry-juice-fights-urinary-tract-infection-quickly.

Yusuf, N. "Photoprotective Effects of Green Tea Polyphenols." *Photodermatology, Photoimmunology & Photomedicine* 23, no. 1 (February 2007): 48–56. http://www.ncbi.nlm.nih.gov/pubmed/17254040.

INDEX

IMAGE CREDITS